The Goddess Diet

The Goddess Diet

Larrian Gillespie

Healthy Life
publications

Visit our website at
http://HEALTHYLIFEPUB.COM

Healthy Life Publications Inc.
264 S. La Cienega Blvd., PMB #1233
Beverly Hills, Calif. 90211
1-800-554-3335
1-310-471-2375
1-310-471-9041 FAX

Publisher's Cataloging-in-Publication
Provided by Quality Books, Inc.
Gillespie, Larrian
        The goddess diet : proven ways to naturally
stay slim, ageless and healthy / Larrian
Gillespie. -- 1st ed.
        p. cm.
        Includes bibliographical references and index.
        LCCN: 99-91469
        ISBN: 0-9671317-3-1

        1. Women--Nutrition. 2. Women--Health and
hygiene. 3.Food--Health aspects. I. Title.

RA778.G55 2000   613.2'082
                          QBI99-1833

First Healthy Life Trade Printing: February 2000

Printed in the U.S.A.

10 9 8 7 6 5 4 3

The information found in this book is from the author's experiences and
is not intended to replace medical advice. The author does not directly or
indirectly dispense medical advice or prescribe the use of this nutritional
program as a form of treatment. This publication is presented for infor-
mational purposes only. Before beginning this or any nutrition program
you should consult with your physician.

Inside cover photo: Robert Cavalli, Still Moving Pictures
Book Design by: Barbara Hoorman
Cover Illustration ©Michael Sullivan, www.artboystudios.com

dedication

To Alexian

Always my daughter
now too my friend

and my mother
Dorothy Olive Gillespie

contents

acknowledgments

A book is never done without the help of so many. I would like to thank Carole Jacobs for burning the midnight oil to edit this book, and Barb Hoorman for her creative styling. I hope you're proud of this book too!

To Elora Alden, for helping me get such a great shape. You make exercising fun!

I have been blessed with so many friends, without whom I may not have made it through many a dark time. To Georganne and Ebar, Cher, Georgia, Emma, Carol and Rosemary, Carol and Mike, Carol and Ray, Carole and Tom, Ali and David, Sharon and Lois, Marilyn and Don, Myra and Alby, Dave and Susan, Lynda and Wayne, CJ, Roy and Gene, Pat, Perry, Lois, Deirdre and Gregg, Annie and Jack, Cate and Cor, Helen and Richard, Helen, Kenn and Joanie, Christian, Gail and Grant, Jim and Anne, Cari and Kyle, Judy and Mike, Bud and Sandy, Fay and Norvel, Meredyth and Shelly, Paula and Gerard, Füsun and Akif, thank you for showing me the meaning of unconditional love.

slim, ageless and healthy

a personal journey

Every woman goes through various changes in her life. At some point, we begin to wonder what really matters in our lives, why we feel the way we do, and why, regardless of how much we "diet" we just can't seem to get rid of those ten (or more) extra pounds. In fact, it seems the more we diet, the more weight we gain. It's enough to make anyone cranky, let alone depressed!

All this had special relevance when it was my figure that began to change as I entered my forties. At first it was gradual, only a few pounds in six months, but within four years I had managed to pack an additional twenty five pounds onto my petite five foot two inch frame. I became an expert at "dress camouflage," emphasizing my newly developed bust line over my ever expanding waistline, while relegating my "older" clothes to the back of the closet. Large, oversize T-shirts substituted as my new uniform while I filled drawers with belts that were no longer "fashionable" for me. What had once been the body of a goddess had now morphed into a spider body—thin arms and legs attached to a large, round torso.

What had once been the body of a goddess had now morphed into a spider body–thin arms and legs attached to a large, round torso

My day of reckoning came when I went for a physical examination and peeked at my report which frankly stated: "white female, mild to moderately obese......" I wanted to scream!!! Me... OBESE!!! I knew what that meant. After all,

I had written it about my very own patients. Obesity was next to slovenliness, carelessness...a glutton. How dare this man write that about me. Didn't he understand it was natural to gain weight when you mature?

The truth hit me hard. I had become obese for my size. As a physician, I was fully aware of the health risks that came with being simply fat. But as someone who enjoyed food and the entire experience of preparing it, I looked forward to dinner, my only real meal of the day. As a surgeon, I skipped breakfast and avoided drinking fluids when I operated so I wouldn't be interrupted by nature's call and there was never enough time for lunch, as patients were waiting in the office. I rationalized every behavior deviation I knew contributed to weight gain, including blaming my mother for making me eat everything on my plate because there were "poor starving children in China." And then I realized if I didn't start putting my own weight loss on the top of my "TO DO" list, I was setting myself up for heart disease, diabetes, hypertension and years of disability.

Women gain and lose weight differently than men

If you would like to understand why all the latest diet herbs, fads, plans and foods simply are not working for you, then come along with me and discover the knowledge and information that can greatly enhance the quality of your life on all levels–physical, mental, emotional and even sexual! This book is about my own personal journey back to being a fit, healthy woman by discovering how women can *naturally* stay slim, ageless and healthy by losing the dangerous abdominal weight ALL of us are prone to gain when our hormones get out of balance. In these chapters, I will em-power you with the ability to avoid this serious health hazard by revealing **why women gain and lose weight differently** than men, supported by the latest scientific research. I will show you why women have been inadvertently fed the wrong information about diet and why we develop a "carbo-hydrate sensitivity syndrome." I will also share with you my perspective on current medical literature so that you can make your own healthy choices about diet and exercise.

Although we need to accept ourselves whether we are "skinny" or "fat" we cannot accept endangering our health by being overweight. The latest longevity stats claim that anyone who reaches the age of 50 by the millennium has a one in two chance of living to 100. With these encouraging odds, no woman can afford to open herself up to the potentially lethal health risks of "letting'er spread". With nearly 55% of American women age 25 and above classified as overweight, obesity has become an epidemic in the United States.[246] Although women live longer than men, they do so with more years of disability.[2]

It's time to own the power of natural health.

chapter one

slim, strong and sensuous

She had the body of a goddess...fit, firm and oozing femininity...while I was dressed as if I had been tented for termites! As I continued to examen my patient, I was reminded of a secret vow I had taken as a young child: never, never to let myself go. No bulging belly...no undulating upper arms that required registration as a lethal weapon...no, I was not going to turn into my great-grandmother!

As a physician who dealt with men and women's reproductive and urinary systems, you would think I'd know how to take proper care of my own body. Unfortunately, doctors are the worst patients. I never exercised, ate the recommended high carbohydrate diet espoused by the AMA, ADA and fashionable fitness magazines and relied upon my great genes to get me through life. And all was well until I turned 40.

I don't want you to think it was something dramatic that happened...far from it. Instead, it was insidious, like grey hair. Actually, I started turning grey, which I blamed on a harrowing episode with a patient who nearly died. Then I noticed my periods, which had always been irregular, were now every 28 days. At the same time, I began to develop an appetite. At first I thought it was just the result of my renewed interest in gourmet cooking, but when I could finish off an entire Lawry's Diamond Jim Brady cut of prime rib, complete with a giant baked potato and salad, I knew something was different.

Until recently, most of the research in muscle metabolism, nutrition and exercise has been conducted using ONLY male participants. So it's no surprise that when the studies were repeated in women, the findings were shockingly different: **while men use carbohydrates for energy, women use them to store as fat.**[3] It seems evolution selected out women who were able to reproduce in the face of starvation, making the female gender extremely efficient at conserving energy. Finally I had the answer to why we could put on pounds simply by breathing in the calories from a chocolate chip cookie!

What I didn't know at the time was the role estrogen played in appetite control

What I didn't know at the time was the role estrogen played in appetite control and our metabolism. Recent research has implicated estradiol, the most potent and active form of estrogen, in the control of eating.[4,5] When estradiol levels drop, so does the release of cholecystokinin, a hormone produced by the pancreas which signals our gallbladders to empty. This in turn makes us feel full or satiated, especially when we have any saturated fat in our diet. But when hormones start to get out of balance, women begin to show a substantial delay in gallbladder emptying and just don't feel full as soon as they should.[6] As a result, portion size increases, and with that the number of calories consumed per feeding.

Changes in our ability to handle carbohydrates add another wallop. As blood sugar rises, so does our hunger quotient and any cholecystokinin released not only fails to signal we're full, but paradoxically increases our appetite.[7] So if you eat a high glycemic carbohydrate, such as popcorn with butter, you'll be even hungrier. Was it any wonder I could eat like a lumberjack! All this made me take a serious look at the changes hormone imbalances were having on my body, especially my stomach. In order to appreciate how different things were becoming, it is important to learn how our digestive system works in the first place.

a trip through your digestive tract

Imagine your stomach is like a washing machine. You first "load" it with food, which has not yet been carefully sorted; that is, proteins, carbohydrates and fat all get tossed in together. Your stomach next adds the "pre-treatment enzymes" and detergent, called hormones. Gastrin stimulates the release of serotonin, histamine, hydrochloric acid and acetylcholine which cause the stomach to contract. The enzyme pepsin efficiently seeks out any of the aromatic amino acids in your food, that is tryptophan, tyrosine and phenylalanine, and chops them off from the rest of the proteins. The "cycle" changes and the emulsified food is now spun into the duodenum, or first part of the small intestine where a concert of actions take place under the direction of the pancreas. First chymotrypsin acts like a "bleach" to remove any residual "stains" or pieces of these same amino acids. At the same time, the pancreas signals your gallbladder to contract by releasing cholecystokinin, which makes you feel full. Carbohydrates and fats are broken down with the help of bile, which is stored in the gallbladder. The pancreas then releases insulin into the bloodstream to handle the sugars that have been extracted from carbohydrates, while the amino acids found in proteins are used to make neurotransmitters. When blood sugar starts to fall too low, the pancreas releases glucagon to prevent hypoglycemia. During all this time, the liver is directing your metabolism based upon the efficiency rating of your digestion. Finally, the pancreas ejects bicarbonate and "rinses" the food, stopping all the action of the stomach's enzymes while it performs the last cycle before sending it to the "dryer", the rest of your small bowel, where any excess water and tiny nutrients left over are absorbed into the bloodstream as the final cleanup from digestion. The entire cycle normally takes about two hours. (Figure 1)

Studies of women experiencing hormone changes, however, show a distinctly different pattern of gastric emptying characterized by prolonged retention of food in the upper or first part of the stomach, preventing the timely release of cholecystokinin. Progesterone is the villain, exerting an antagonistic effect on the gastric nerves. Falling estrogen levels lead to complaints of an upset stomach and heartburn as excess progesterone relaxes the lower esophageal sphincter. This is especially noticeable at night, as lying flat in bed allows acid to

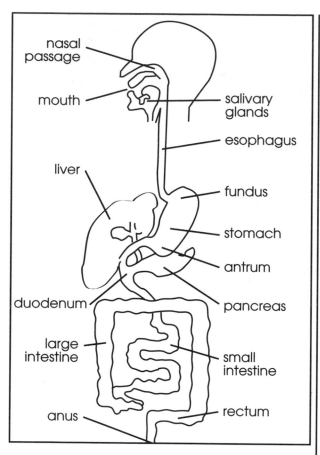

nasal
passage

mouth

salivary
glands

esophagus

liver

fundus

stomach

antrum

duodenum

pancreas

large
intestine

small
intestine

anus

rectum

figure 1
*the digestive
system*

flow back out of the stomach, irritating the esophagus.

Not only does our stomach fail to empty on time, but this change in our digestion starts a domino effect on metabolism. Distension of the stomach occurs which sends stretch signals to nerves surrounding the bottom of the stomach. The gallbladder, in response, becomes sluggish, and doesn't empty completely. This prevents the complete emulsification of fats in our diet. When we eat cereals, oils, sugars and meat instead of fish and fruits, we predispose ourselves to develop gallstones.[8] In a study of Italians, women who eat a low carbohydrate, high fiber diet and avoid alcohol have the least risk of developing gallstones.[9] A diet which limits calories to less than 2500 a day, decreases saturated fat and carbohydrates greatly reduces the risk of gallstones.[10]

The efficiency of our duodenal enzymes to break down food properly is compromised when our hormones start to change. As a result, our intestines are forced to handle incompletely digested particles, which exposes their delicate surface to damaging agents, called free radicals. These atoms of highly-reactive oxygen bombard healthy cells like meteors, and knock through their protective surfaces. Free radicals are also introduced into the body by certain foods, tobacco smoke, air and water. As they roam throughout the body, they bind to and change the structure of cell membranes, making them "leaky", which prematurely ages a cell. Soon your tissue becomes acidotic and the cell ceases to function normally. This intracellular warfare can even damage blood vessels so that atherosclerotic plaques build up on the ragged surface. All this can lead to inflammation, irritable bowel syndrome and even cancer.

It is not surprising that the stomachs of women who are experiencing hormone imbalances react more severely when infected with Helicobacter pylori, the infectious bacteria responsible for ulcers. While females with normal hormone balance are able to keep their immune reaction to a low level, women with lower estrogen levels demonstrate weeping, destructive inflammation of the fundus (first part) of the stomach and the antrum (lower part).[11] The delayed emptying allows the bacteria to remain in contact with the tissue for a longer period of time, increasing its virulence. Without the ability to properly stimulate the release of cholecystokinin another hormone, somatostatin, is not produced to protect the stomach lining.[12] Like magic, you've created an ulcer.

Free radicals make cell membranes "leaky" which prematurely ages a cell

our bodies not ourselves

If I'm honest with you, the ten years before we stop menstruating are the toughest on our bodies. As I told a patient, "Once the ovaries are dead, its easy. It's the dying that's the hard part!" There were days I swore my ovaries were threatening suicide. So let's look at the "risk factors" for causing your periods to stop.

In a study performed in Sweden, about 500 women who had been without a period for one year were studied.[13] Any woman who had a surgical or medical reason for not having a period was excluded. Their findings were significant. The more a woman smokes the younger she will be when her periods stop. This is linked with a lower lung capacity, causing them to have less oxygen in their blood than their non-smoker associates. These same women also reported a higher degree of tiredness. It makes sense that if you can't get oxygen to the tissue, you'll cause cells to age more rapidly and die quicker. An anti-estrogenic effect of smoking has been suggested though the mechanism is not understood. What is clear is that women smokers have less body fat, and that affects the blood levels of estrogens, which raises cholesterol and accelerates the aging process. But these are not the only interesting discoveries. The ability to continue menstruating is connected with a higher serum insulin and uric acid level. In fact, at the age of 40, a high insulin level is considered a marker for normal female sex hormone function and NOT for insulin resistance, as seen in post-menopausal women. So what does this mean? As we age, our bodies begin to develop a sensitivity to carbohydrates as our estrogen levels start to fall, around the age of 40. To understand the significance of this, let me explain what insulin has to do with our ability to metabolize carbohydrates.

A diet which limits calories to less than 2500 a day, decreases saturated fat and carbohydrates greatly reduces the risk of gallstones

carbohydrate sensitivity syndrome

Let's start with a normal, ovulating female, that is, someone usually around 30 (remember, like everything, there are two ends to the bell curve and some women can be stop ovulating at 35). Carbohydrates are divided into two categories: complex and simple. It is perhaps easiest to think of these foods as starches and sugars which vary in the size of their particles. A simple carbohydrate has very small, fine particles, like sugar or refined, processed foods while complex carbs are more like raw, natural, large molecules such as, lentils, squash and broccoli. In the course of "normal" digestion, it takes longer to absorb most large molecules because all food has to be broken down into the smallest particle. That is why small, simple carbohydrates get into your blood stream the fastest. However, some complex carbohydrates contain more natural sugar and can be quicker to get into the blood, such as corn, acting like a simple carbohydrate in triggering your body's insulin response.

Glucose is the fuel which enables the mitochondria to act like a thermonuclear reactor, splitting off electrons which generate energy for cellular function. Most importantly, every organ in our body requires glucose to function. Glucose is either used immediately as your cell's energy source or stored in the form of glycogen in the liver and in muscle as emergency reserves. Once these sites are full, the rest is stored as fat.

The role of insulin is to keep blood glucose levels from rising too high by shoving glucose, amino acids and free fatty acids from the bloodstream as quickly as possible into every cell for immediate use. Like a teeter-totter glucagon, another hormone, prevents insulin from being too efficient and causing hypoglycemia. Both hormones are secreted by the pancreas. When we eat carbohydrates, the petite particles are absorbed from the small intestine into our bloodstream and we have an elevated glucose level. Like the newest vacuum cleaner, insulin "beats, it sweeps, it cleans" our blood of glucose by shoving it into cells, then storing any excess in fat cells. As if to add insult to injury, insulin signals previously stored fat to stay put while excess free fatty acids are then sent to the liver where they are converted into cholesterol. Remember, hormones are the chemical internet within your body that directs the breakdown and buildup of new cells. When estrogen levels are low or out of balance, insulin levels go up and that leads to more cells breaking down, giving us that haggard look of accelerated aging.

Glucagon, on the other hand, is stimulated by proteins and a lowering glucose level and has the laudable job of promoting the breakdown of stored fat in order to achieve equilibrium. This is a GOOD thing! It's also capable of aiding the liver in converting amino acids derived from protein into glucose in case of starvation. The exciting news is that once glucagon levels are elevated, they remain so for at least four hours.[14]

hormone-dependent changes

As you can tell, our bodies undergo a lot of changes when our hormones are out of balance, the most significant of which may be alteration in our sensitivity to insulin. As estrogen decreases, thyroid levels begin to drop while insulin loses its effectiveness in lowering our blood sugar. This causes our pancreas to have to work overtime putting out more than the usual amount of insulin to do the same job. You already know that insulin aids in storing fat. This makes it MORE efficient at storing the excess glucose as fat as it becomes LESS efficient at lowering our blood glucose levels. An increase in body mass occurs. In short...we develop a carbohydrate sensitivity syndrome (CSS) and we start to become fat. In fact, a specific syndrome, called Metabolic Syndrome X, has been identified in women. It is characterized by women who have two or more of the following conditions: insulin resistance with resulting elevated insulin levels, elevated lipids (especially triglycerides), obesity, coronary artery disease and hypertension. Not surprisingly, it has been found to be associated with estrogen deficiency.[15,16]

Lower estrogen levels not only prevent ovulation but affect another hormone, serotonin, which is important in controlling our mood. When you eat a low protein, low fat diet, you deprive the brain of the ability to make serotonin, which can result in depression and even headaches. More importantly, low serotonin levels signal the thyroid to slow down your metabolism. Stress and high carbohydrate diets add to this pyramid of hormonal imbalances. Prescriptions for selective serotonin-reuptake inhibitors, such as Prozac and Zoloft, have reached epidemic proportions in women because we are depriving our bodies of the best building materials in our diet—protein.

Statistics indicate that 34% of white women, almost

50% of African American women and 48% of Hispanic women are overweight.[1] Obesity is responsible for hypertension, gallstones, endometrial, kidney and breast cancer, heart attacks and diabetes, just to name a few diseases that can be modified or even prevented by losing as little as 5-10 pounds.[17-23] As women, we simply can't afford to trivialize the impact obesity has on our health.

Until now, women have been treated like men when it comes to dietary advice. As a result, we have failed to follow our intuition when it comes to choosing foods that harmonize with our hormones. So, if you're ready to unleash the healthy, ageless goddess within each and every one of you by improving your metabolism and achieving your ideal body composition, let me show you the factors **uniquely designed for women** which form an essential part in making us naturally slim, strong and sensuous!

Obesity is responsible for hypertension, gallstones, endometrial, kidney and breast cancer, heart attacks and diabetes

chapter two

buddha belly syndrome: the hidden danger

Scientists are only now discovering that a healthy weight is not defined by the numbers on a scale, but by where fats are stored in the body. More importantly, not all fat cells behave alike, with the most metabolically active ones hiding like some creature in the dark deep inside the abdomen. As a result, you can be simultaneously very fit but fairly fat. Genetics plays a role in this, but scientists are acknowledging that our hormone balance dictates where women put on fat.

fat's gotten under your skin

Both visceral and subcutaneous fat have the same composition—75% fatty acids and 25% glycerol, a type of alcohol. While the fat cells inside our abdomen are smaller than their distant cousins on our hips, these little creatures are more active, releasing fatty acids into the blood stream while picking up additional fat for storage. Because they can snuggle up to the blood vessels surrounding all our internal organs, they can deliver fatty acids to tissue with little constraint. This means the liver is bathed with blood that is very high in free fatty acids, which results in less of the good cholesterol, called high density lipoproteins (HDL) and more of the bad or low density cholesterol (LDL). Any tissue surrounded by fatty acids is less able to remove insulin from the bloodstream, which results in increased fat storage. The more intra-abdominal fat, the higher the insulin levels.[24]

the omentum

As a surgeon, I constantly encountered the omentum, a fatty apron of tissue that performs the function of a barrier between the lining of the abdomen and the bowel in order to prevent adhesions. This organ acts as a giant sponge within your abdomen soaking up any fluid in contact with it...blood, electrolyte solutions, lymph or fluid from ovarian cysts. It has the additional ability to concentrate neurochemicals, especially norepinephrine, epinephrine and dopamine from the GI tract in its venous blood and tissue.[25] This makes it a very active biological organ, capable of mobilizing fat in response to insulin and cortisol. This organ is able to swell and enlarge when faced with excess amounts of these neurotransmitters, which are found in red meat and manufactured from foods high in the amino acids tryptophan, tyrosine and tyramine. If you've ever eaten a meal and felt the uncomfortable tug of your belt before you left the table, it's your omentum working overtime. (Figure 2)

The more intra-abdominal fat, the higher the insulin levels

the rules of fat distribution

The regulation of fat distribution is a highly complex process, entailing profound effects on metabolism. By measuring the turnover of fat tissue triglycerides, researchers were able to show that fats are first stored in the omentum and retroperitoneal areas (the deep parts of your pelvis), then the subcutaneous regions of the abdomen and finally in the subcutaneous femoral area on the thigh.[26] In pre-menopausal women subcutaneous abdominal fat has a higher turnover than femoral fat tissue, a difference that disappears with menopause and is restored by estrogen. With abdominal fat, multiple hormone changes are found including elevated cortisol and male sex hormones in women, due to the information highway connecting the hypothalamus, pituitary and adrenals. Adrenaline is a protein utilizing hormone which can waste away your lean muscle mass and increase your insulin resistance. The more muscle cells you deplete, the less storage sites for sugar. Fat

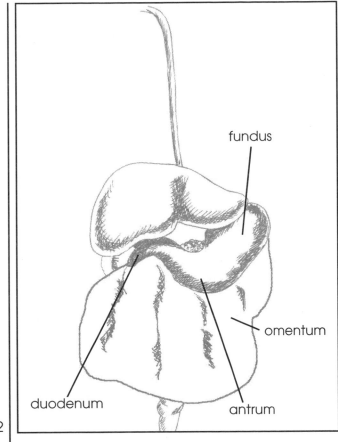

figure 2

cells, under the direction of cortisol and insulin, promote fat storage by expressing lipoprotein lipase, a fat accumulating enzyme. Abdominal fat cells pack more in per square inch, and have a greater blood supply along with more nerve connections to detour fats to their area. In short, the balance between the fat accumulating couple (cortisol and insulin) and the fat mobilizing couple (estrogen and growth hormone) is shifted in favor of the former in menopause, polycystic ovarian syndrome, aging, depression, stress, chronic dieting, smoking and excess alcohol intake.

location location location

Like real estate, everything about fat boils down to its location. Fat cells, called adipocytes, have limits on how much fat they can store dependent upon their position in the body. Intra-abdominal or visceral cells are the sumo wrestlers of fat storage, enlarging to gargantuan size when we put our bodies under chronic stress. These lard buckets have more receptors for glucocorticoids than peripheral fat cells, allowing them to preferentially direct the fat traffic to their sites.[27] Insulin causes fluid retention by making us more sensitive to salt and expands the tissue surrounding these cells. Cortisol speeds up the intestine's ability to transport fat and this makes it harder for fat depots to clear out glycerol and free fatty acids, the products of fat breakdown, which prevents further mobilization of fat.[28] You can almost hear those fat cells squishing when you chomp down on a "stress relieving" bag of potato chips.

Insulin causes fluid retention by making us more sensitive to salt and expands the tissue surrounding these cells

the sensitive side of fat

Abdominal fat has a significantly stronger relationship with insulin sensitivity than peripheral non-abdominal fat, making women with the Spider Body shape more insulin resistant than those with fat on their thighs.[24] Scientists say abdominal fat may be a major reason why women develop insulin resistance.

With central obesity there is an increased risk for breast and endometrial cancer due to elevated levels of circulating estrogens created from alterations of male sex steroids or androgens in fat tissue combined with decreased levels of sex hormone-binding globulin (SHBG).[29] As insulin levels go up, the ovaries increase the production of male sex hormones—testosterone and androstenedione—and infertility occurs.[30,31] Meals high in carbohydrates stimulate higher levels of insulin which in turn causes a rise in androgens. Obese women with infertility are probably stimulating their disease process with every meal they eat. The great news is all this can be reversed by simply losing weight.[32]

The bad news is even a normal weight can be

unhealthy in some women. Scientists measured the hidden fat within the abdomen of normal weight women by computerized tomography, or a CAT scan. Using a body mass index (BMI) of 25 as normal, they were able to determine that women aged 40 and above who had not completed menopause should have a desirable waist measurement less than 31 1/2 inches. A healthy goddess has a waist less than 26 inches, and if you are post-menopausal, you should strive for less than 29 1/2 inches if you don't want to raise your risk factors for heart disease and diabetes.[33] The swing of the needle on a scale means very little if you stuff your abdomen with most of your fat.[24]

the chinese connection

The significance of this information crosses all cultural lines. Studies on healthy Chinese men and women who had heavy upper bodies were at a higher risk of cardiovascular disease even though they weren't technically fat.[34] Deep intra-abdominal fat correlated with higher blood pressure, glucose, triglyceride and low HDL levels — all known to put us at increased risk for heart disease. So even eating a traditional oriental diet can't change the impact central body fat has on our survival. After reading this research, I knew I could no longer justify the "Buddha Belly" I had acquired. My father died of a sudden, unexpected heart attack and his parents and brothers as well. I had inherited their body shape and genetics, but I was determined to prevent my genes from controlling my destiny.

how body shape can predict health problems

All women are NOT created equal when it comes to the shape of our bodies, as anyone knows whose stood in the open changing room at Loehmann's. Some women are pear shaped, with "saddle bag" thighs and buttocks, while others carry most of their "pot" on the belly and upper hips. But did you know that where you put on fat is directly under the control of your hormones?

hormones: fat dictators

During our childbearing years, estrogen directs fat to be stored on our hips and thighs as a quick access site for energy during breast-feeding. Physicians refer to this shape as a "gynecoid" or feminine figure. (Figure 3A) Once our estrogen levels start to drop, we no longer prefer our legs as storage sites for fat and we start hoarding blubber under the skin and within the abdomen. This gives us a different body shape, called "android", which makes us look more like a man. (Figure 3B) This change is brought about by age, plain and simple. Growth hormone, which directs our fat metabolism and helps to build muscles, takes an elevator ride to the basement and we start to lose fat burning muscle mass. Once this happens our ability to burn calories falls and any excess food that finds its way down our digestive tracts gets sidelined into fat.[16,35] As we replace lean muscle with fat, we keep lowering our energy efficiency rating. Total body weight goes up and that's when the problems really start.

Hormones rule our bodies. I know you don't like to hear this but it's true. The amazing part is how

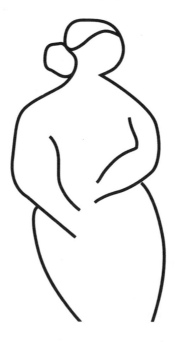

figure 3A
*gynecoid
shape*

something as simple as fat can start a chain reaction that will send our entire bodies spiraling into hormone hell.

insulin: the evil twin

When we gain fat a not-so-funny thing happens to our insulin levels – they go up – and that results in more fat storage. It seems insulin can act like an evil twin, lowering our blood sugar when present in small amounts (the GOOD twin) but let it hang around for a while and it turns us into porkers. Progesterone, another hormone that helps us to hold onto a pregnancy in our fertile years, stimulates the pancreas to secrete insulin, and the more insulin in circulation, the more hostile our tissue becomes to its action of lowering glucose in our blood.[36,37] Cholesterol levels go up and the concentration of the good triglycerides goes down. High, sustained insulin levels accelerate the formation of blood clots, and that makes us more susceptible to strokes and heart attacks. As a final kick in the pants, it stiffens our blood vessels, causing hypertension.

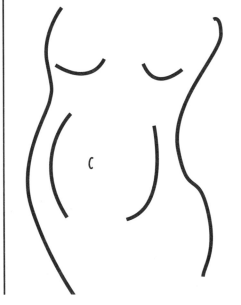

figure 3B
*android
shape*

the apple and the pear:
it's not the garden of eden

So how do you tell if you have an apple or pear shaped body? The most reliable indicator seems to be your waist-to-hip ratio (WHR) followed by the circumference of your waist. To find your WHR, measure around the fullest part of your buttocks (this is your hip measurement) and then measure your waist (the narrowest part of your torso between your lowest rib and your iliac crest or hip bone.) Simply divide your waist by your hip measurement. A healthy ratio is less than .8 with an ideal ratio around .74. A WHR greater than 0.85 is characteristic of upper body obesity. Women with this android or male body shape have more bloated fat cells, higher sustained insulin levels, which become less effective at lowering their blood sugar, and are often producing large amounts of male sex hormones. In addition, they have elevated plasma lipid profiles and are at a high risk of developing non-insulin dependent diabetes.[38]

According to a study published in JAMA, women with a WHR of 0.76 or higher or a waist circumference of 30 inches or greater have more than a 2-fold higher risk of coronary heart disease.[39] Further studies show that women who gain weight in their abdomen have a higher risk of developing heart disease than those who gain weight in their legs.[40] So what is directing all these changes? A wedge-shaped gland called the hypothalamus.

High, sustained insulin levels accelerate the formation of blood clots, and that makes us more susceptible to strokes and heart attacks

this is your brain on patrol

Located at the base of the third ventricle in the brain, the hypothalamus acts as the "Great and Wonderful Wizard" of our hormones sending signals to the pituitary which in turn shouts orders to the other endocrine glands – the adrenals, thyroid and ovaries. (Figure 4) As our supply of eggs decreases, information is sent back to the hypothalamus informing it of an upcoming shortage in estrogen. This makes it a little hypersensitive – okay, plain cranky – and it begins to order the adrenal glands to swell, or hypertrophy in order to produce an alternate pathway for estrogen production. Once the adrenals swing into action cortisol, the stress hormone, gets released and fat cells open up to take on more storage. The amount of fat metabolism changes dramatically and those fat cells which have a greater blood supply turn into gluttons. Unfortunately, these are the very ones that surround the bowel and line our abdominal cavity giving us the android shape.

the threat to your health

Diabetes strikes over 8 million people, while an additional 8 million remain undiagnosed with non-insulin dependent diabetes (NIDDM or type II).[41] Astonishingly, an estimated 20 million persons meet the criteria for impaired glucose tolerance, a condition in which blood glucose levels are higher than normal but not high enough to be diagnosed as diabetes. Hyperglycemia and impaired glucose tolerance, as seen when our hormones get out of balance, convey a significant risk for heart disease and full-blown diabetes.[42] Not surprisingly, it's the sugar extracted by our stomach from the foods we eat that results in the high glucose levels seen after eating in early undiagnosed diabetes. In fact, the first sign of diabetes is elevated glucose for several hours after a meal.[43]

Women who gain weight in their abdomen have a higher risk of developing heart disease than those who gain weight in their legs

Coronary artery disease kills more women, nearly 500,000 annually, than all cancers combined.[44] Women with heart disease are also more likely to suffer from diabetes, hypertension and high cholesterol levels than men. After menopause, the chance of dying from a heart attack in women nearly equals those of men. A postmenopausal woman has a 31% lifetime mortality risk from heart disease in contrast to a 2.8% risk of dying from a hip fracture or breast cancer.[45] As many as 1 in 8 women aged 45 to 54 has clinical evidence of heart disease. It seems cholesterol numbers can be deceiving. Excess sugar can result in cholesterol being deposited as a liquid plaque within the blood vessels feeding the heart, especially in women. This type of

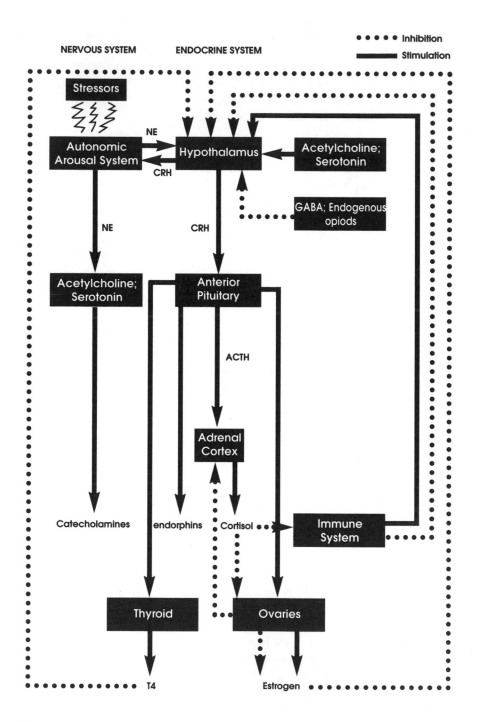

figure 4

plaque doesn't block the vessels like a column, and can't be detected by treadmills or angiograms. Not surprisingly, the formation of these liquid filled cavities is aggrevated by elevated insulin levels. Once they burst, they fill the entire blood vessel with a core of cholesterol, making them a silent killer in women with hormonal imbalances. You've probably already guessed the two most significant risk factors for developing either diabetes or heart disease-smoking and abdominal obesity.

and now for the buddha belly awards

So what are the risk factors for gaining abdominal or central fat? In a study done by the American Cancer Society, women who eat large amounts of saturated fat, especially from meat, frequently drink alcohol, smoke, have multiple pregnancies or have gained a lot of weight since the age of 18 have twice as much chance of winning the "Buddha Belly Award" than women who eat a diet high in vegetables, exercise, or take estrogen faithfully if they are menopausal.[46]

Gaining weight does more than make you look fat— it can endanger your health, shorten your life span and even trigger life-threatening diseases. Now for the good news. If you look at all the illnesses listed in Table 1, each and every one can be modified by losing that unhappy Buddha Belly.

If you're ready to change your lifestyle and want to be healthy and fit for the rest of your life, let me show you how simple it is to lose the weight and keep it off. You don't need pills or surgery and you can end up saving a lot of money. Interested? Then let's get started.

Table 1

---

buddha belly damage factors

- Arthritis
- Hypertension
- Cancer of the breast, endometrium, kidneys
- Incontinence
- Coronary Heart Disease
- Kidney failure
- Chronic lung disease
- Kidney stones
- Diabetes
- Polycystic ovarian disease
- Gallstones
- Sleep apnea
- Stroke
- Irritable Bowel Syndrome
- Migraines
- Depression
- Infertility
- Osteoporosis
- Bloating
- PMS
- Cataracts

chapter three

the goddess diet

It seems like your worst nightmare. After days of dieting and yes, even starvation, you sneak up on the bathroom scale like a stealth bomber only to discover you're still no thinner! According to Prevention, the world's largest health magazine, weight gain is the number one complaint of women.[47] How food affects hormones is the focus of dietary endocrinology and scientists are only now starting to assess why women gain and lose weight differently than men.

It's a scientific fact. Women's stomachs respond differently than men's when digesting a meal. Numerous studies agree that we take almost an hour longer than men to empty our stomachs due to the effect of progesterone on the motility of the antrum, or lower portion of the stomach.[48] As a result, we are much more efficient at grabbing every little bit of carbohydrate from the foods we eat before we digest protein and fat.[49] This causes a more sustained rise in insulin, which increases our ability to store fat. In fact, our blood insulin and glucose levels can stay high for up to five hours after a 500 to 1000 calorie meal. This can set the stage for heart disease, hypertension, obesity, cataracts and the signs of aging.

This delayed but prolonged rise in insulin and glucose in response to carbohydrates inhibits the release of glucagon, the hormone that helps us to burn previously stored fat. In normal people, (they mean men...bear with me) within thirty minutes of eating protein, glucagon levels start to rise, peaking at two hours.[50] In fact, glucagon can stay elevated in blood for several hours after a protein rich meal. This gives your body plenty of time to use the fat around your waist and hips as the energy source to fuel your brain.

all carbohydrates are not created equal

Since 1927, scientists have known that different carbohydrates with the same nutrient composition produce different glucose responses in the body.[51] A "sugar profile" was developed for each food enabling doctors to predict the effect of digestion on the availability of glucose in the body. By comparing other foods to the glucose response which you achieve by eating just a few slices of white bread, a glycemic index of carbohydrate metabolism was established.[52-54] This gave doctors the freedom to exchange carbohydrate choices for diabetic patients without risking big swings in their blood glucose levels.

Women's stomachs respond differently than men's when digesting a meal

Not all foods, however, are created equal. The particle size of a particular food and the degree of gelatinization which it undergoes when cooked affects how much glucose or sugar can be obtained by digestion. Rice is a good example of a food that can vary markedly depending upon the amylose content. The higher the amylose, the greater the gelatinization and the lower the glycemic index (GI).[55] The more processed a food becomes, the smaller the particle size and the greater the GI. That's why bread, french fries, corn chips, canned pea soup, angel food cake and Cheerios™ have almost identical GI values and insulin responses.[56]

the uniqueness of women

When it comes to measuring blood glucose responses, women are definitely unique. A standard glucose tolerance test extends over 2-4 hours, while in diabetic patients and women with carbohydrate sensitivity syndrome (CSS), 3-5 hours are needed to get a complete profile.[57,58] All this has to do with the rate of digestion. Like diabetics, women add an additional hour onto digestion because they are unable to move food from the bottom or antral portion due to delays in activating the sympathetic nerves which stimulate the stomach to empty. As a result, women and diabetics have a slower rise in the glucose and insulin response to food and these levels can remain slightly above fasting for several hours.[59] Since our bodies were designed to feed "two" this was a very handy adaptation. However, once our periods stop, it becomes a handicap.

protein power

Much has been made about the ability of protein to decrease blood sugar levels when added to a carbohydrate meal. The exact effect, however, depends upon both the type and amount of protein and the medical condition of the person eating the combination. In normal people (remember that's a man by scientific definition) and non-insulin dependent diabetics (NIDDM) protein stimulates insulin secretion but not glucose, which causes a drop in blood sugar. However, it requires a LOT of protein to do this. Let me give you an example: Four slices of white bread contain 50 gm of carbohydrate which acts like 3 tablespoons of corn syrup in your body. It would take 50 gm of protein or 12 ounces or 3 chicken breasts to cause a drop in blood sugar in response to eating that bread.[60] If you were an insulin-dependent diabetic, you would increase rather than decrease your blood sugar levels by adding that much protein to your meal.

Protein, however, does stimulate the production of glucagon which, along with cholecystokinin, can help to decrease your meal size by signaling that you're full.[61] When protein is eaten first, it stimulates glucagon and the hormone motilin, which jump starts the gastric wave to empty the stomach.

Women add an additional hour onto digestion

fat facts

Fat, especially saturated fat, slows down the rate at which your stomach is able to process foods. In addition, it also impedes the activity of the small bowel in propelling food along your digestive tract.[62] Delayed gastric emptying will have the effect of lowering your blood sugar response to a meal. A lot has been made about eating specific ratios of fat and protein in order to maintain normal glucose levels. This Zone approach is not in line with current research. If you put 25 gms of fat or 2 1/2 tablespoons of butter on white bread it will have no effect on preventing the sugar rise in normal people.[63] The addition of fat to a carbohydrate gives you the same blood sugar response as if you ate the carbohydrate alone but a greater insulin response. This is not good, as the longer insulin stays around, the more hostile your tissue becomes to letting go of fat. So it seems fat and protein, when added to a meal, can reduce your blood sugar response but only if relatively large amounts of either are used.[64]

Eating a breakfast full of low glycemic carbs can lower your insulin response

mix it up

When you eat a "mixed meal" of protein, carbohydrate and fat, the amount of blood sugar rise can be predicted from the glycemic index of the carbohydrate alone. This is significant, because only by choosing foods that are low in their ability to turn your body into a sugar cube can you achieve a more normal insulin response.[65] Furthermore, by eating a breakfast full of low glycemic carbs you can lower your insulin response to a standard lunch meal by as much as 30%.[66] An added benefit of eating low GI foods is a normal bowel movement, as nearly 20% of the undigested starch from these foods will be metabolized in the colon, acting as additional fiber in your diet.

graze or gorge

Another way to keep your blood sugar under control is to eat frequent small meals instead of one big meal. Snacking on 250 calorie "mini meals" can keep your insulin levels down, which in turn lowers your cholesterol.[58] As an added bonus, small meals relieve the stress on your body, as evidenced by lower cortisol and cholesterol levels and make it easier for your stomach to empty.[67,68] By simply reducing the rate at which you present food to your digestive tract you can dramatically reduce the rate of lipids or fats appearing in your blood regardless of what you eat.

Are you a gorger who eats most of your calories at one meal? If you are, the saturated fat and high glycemic carbohydrates in that meal packs a whollop. You essentially overload the circuitry of your body's digestive process and cause a "blackout" which has devastating effects on your circulation, not to mention your waistline. But if you snack on 5 to 7 meals a day with the same amount of calories, you maintain an even, smooth level of sugar and fats in your blood. Your electric grid stays lit without any signs of overload. By spreading the calories of a meal throughout the course of a day your body will trigger a counter regulatory mechanism that sends growth hormone levels up for 4 hours after each meal. Remember, the more growth hormone around, the more you burn fat, not muscle.

Our bodies can tolerate a rise in fat levels between 10 to 30% and still keep the insulin, glucose and corticosterone levels low, but if we eat more than 30% fat at a single sitting we end up with elevated blood sugar levels and more fat storage.[69] By eating mini meals and spreading the calories, our bodies can handle a fat load in excess of 30% and still not lose control.[70]

can one meal affect the next?

Our bodies can be downright stingy when it comes to letting insulin out of the vault if we eat meals closer together. Known as the Staub-Traugott effect, scientists have shown the closeness of one meal to the next determines the blood sugar response to the following meal; the closer together the meals are, the better the glucose tolerance and the less insulin the body needs to keep your blood sugar in check.

The amount of fiber in a meal can also affect the burst of insulin you release when faced with the next meal. Fiber, by its sheer ability to slow down digestion, can lower blood glucose levels. High fiber soups can significantly suppress hunger and reduce the amount of calories desired in the next meal, especially if you eat a "chunky" soup.[71] But this is not the main reason the composition of one meal affects the next one's ability to raise your blood sugar. In a study of mixed meals with different fiber contents but the same glycemic carbohydrate content, researchers found that a dinner composed of low glycemic carbohydrates improved your carbohydrate tolerance for breakfast.[72] It's like having an overdraft built into your carbohydrate checkbook.

the french paradox

Now that you understand the advantages of "mini meals" you have understood a paradigm that stumped researchers for years, called The French Paradox. It seems our French relations, who helped us win our independence from England, may also be helping us lose the fat. Although the French eat a higher saturated fat diet, smoke and drink alcohol, they have 40% fewer heart attacks than Americans.

So how do they do it?

- The French are consumers of moderate amounts of alcohol, especially red wine, usually with meats

- The French eat more fresh fruit and vegetables

- The French eat less red meat

- The French consume more cheese and less whole milk

- The French use more olive oil and less butter or lard, and they take longer to eat meals and snack less on high carbohydrate foods

Now, not all things are good for all people, as you will see with wine. However, there are several important points to remember. Eating a diet high in fruit and vegetables offers your body high levels of folate, which lowers plasma homocysteine levels. Even mild to moderate elevation in blood values of this amino acid is a strong risk factor for atherosclerosis clogging up arteries to the brain, heart and limbs.[73] In a study of diet diversity and quality of the French, researchers found that few French adults consumed diets consistent with the American USDA recommendations. Only 14% of those studied got their fat levels below 30% and less than 4% consumed less than 10% of that as saturated fat. In contrast, 90% of them had the most diverse diet, with women choosing more "vitamin dense" foods, while those who did meet the USDA requirements scored the lowest in food choices.[74,75] Much like the advice given by any financial advisor, diversity in your food choices seems to be an important factor in protecting your life's assets against fluctuations in the energy consumption market.

Although the French are not known for their exercise clubs, their lifestyles are naturally more active. They live in small villages where they walk and their lives don't revolve around cars and malls. They shop and carry home fresh food daily and rarely prepare meals from the cupboard. Foods are available seasonally, not year round which affects the nutritional content of the food. Cars are a luxury, necessitating several episodes of walking per day with weighted packages. Meals in restaurants are expensive, so more socialization is done at wine bars or bistros where a single dish can be consumed over an hour of friendly conversation. But most of all the French understand the importance of breakfast, especially among women with low BMI or body mass index.[76] They are more aware of the importance of choosing foods that offer protection against heart disease and cancer. Eating fruits and vegetables, especially tomatoes, can protect against cancers of the digestive and respiratory tracts.[77,78] French women who are obese eat more like Americans. They don't eat breakfast, consume only three meals a day and spend more time watching television.[79,80]

The French understand the importance of breakfast

fudging with fat

Numerous studies have reported a positive link between dietary fat and fatness. However, only recently have researchers focused on the type of fat in addition to the quantity in our diets. It seems fat intake can only explain about 2% of the fat snuggled under your skin and hiding in your abdomen.[81] In a study specifically of pre and postmenopausal women, including African Americans, changes in the amount of saturated fat intake had a dramatic effect on lowering cholesterol, especially LDL or the bad low density cholesterol.[82] When another group of postmenopausal women were placed on a 26% fat diet consisting of 14% monounsaturated fats with only 6% saturated fat, they too improved their cholesterol profiles.[83] It seems fudging your fat intake by substituting more mono-unsaturated fats like olive oil can result not only in weight loss but a much better cholesterol and insulin response.[84] Even a handful of peanuts, which are rich in oleic acid can make a difference in a women's risk for heart disease.[85]

Butter doesn't deserve the bad rep it's gotten when it comes to the effect of different fats on cholesterol levels in your blood, liver and gallbladder. While palm, coconut and olive oil caused the highest concentration of cholesterol in the blood, butter produced an intermediate response in all three categories and was not

Table 4

dietary sources of essential fatty acids

Fatty Acid	Food source	Enriched source
Linoleic acid	vegetable oils	corn oil
Alpha linolenic acid	seeds, nuts	black currant oil flaxseed
Gamma linolenic acid	seeds, nuts	primrose borage oil
Arachidonic acid	red meat	
Eicosapentaenoic acid	seafood	fish oil
Docosahexaenoic acid	seafood	fish oil

linked to gallstone formation.[86] Butter also contains buteric acid, which helps you absorb nutrients from your food. So don't be afraid to incorporate unsalted butter into your diet if you're watching your cholesterol.

digging your grave with your own teeth

Unfortunately, all these facts fly in the face of the very diet your doctor or other experts may be suggesting. The current recommended diet for women emphasizes substituting carbohydrates for saturated fat without concern for their ability to raise your blood sugar level. No wonder women are going nuts trying to figure out why they are gaining weight![87] Low fat, high carbohydrate diets increase the insulin concentration in your blood, which can raise your risk for heart disease. The more insulin resistant you become, the greater will be the negative effects on insulin, glucose and cholesterol if you consume a high carbohydrate, low fat diet. Studies bear this out.

Two diets were tested using the following composition of carbohydrates, fat and protein: Group 1

Table 5

Low fat, high carbohydrate diets increase the insulin concentration in your blood, which can raise your risk for heart disease

diseases promoted by fat

- Coronary heart disease
- Stroke
- Stomach cancer
- Colon cancer
- Pancreatic cancer
- Prostate cancer
- Breast cancer
- Ovarian cancer
- Endometrial cancer

ate a 60/25/15 ratio and Group 2 consumed a 40/45/15 diet. That's right—45% fat. The ratio of mono/poly and saturated fat were the same. As predicted, those who substituted carbs for fat had a marked decrease in the good high density cholesterol with an overall elevation in LDL /HDL ratios to above 4, which is considered dangerous.[88-90] This is not an isolated study, but rather consistent with numerous large epidemiological studies of women and their risk for heart disease.[91-94] The answer seems clear: low fat, high carbohydrate diets can cause dangerous changes in your health, especially if you are insulin resistant. It's like digging your own grave with your teeth every time you load up on high glycemic carbs. It just makes sense to decrease the saturated fat in your diet by increasing the amount of mono-unsaturated fats and low glycemic carbs instead of reaching for that potato. And if you want to maintain your weight loss, monounsaturated fatty acids are the key.[83] (Table 4) Trouble letting go of saturated fats? Do as I did—decrease the frequency rather than the quantity at a given meal.

fat and cancer

Everyone's blaming fats for causing cancer. Just look at the diseases listed in Table 5. While saturated fat can increase your risk, there is little evidence that monounsaturated fats affect tumors. As the American public decreased their consumption of butter and dairy, they substituted n-6-polyunsaturated oils-vegetable oils-which unfortunately have a very strong cancer promoting effect. (Table 6) As a result, there has been a direct increase in the incidence of postmenopausal breast cancer. The higher concentration of fats and phospholipids as well as increased levels of estrogen produced from the conversion of body fat to estradiol is to blame. No greater proof of the association between high dietary fat and breast cancer need be provided than to look at the current rise in diseases related to dietary fats in countries like Japan and even our own 50th State Hawaii.[19,95] An intake of 40% or more of fat leads to this effect, which can be reduced by dropping the amount of saturated fat.[96]

Table 6

oils and their composition of fats

Oil	PU	MU	Total Unsat	Sat
Olive	9	77	86	14
Canola	36	58	94	6
Peanut	34	48	82	18
Corn	62	25	87	13
Soybean	61	24	85	15
Sunflower	77	14	91	9
Safflower	77	14	91	9
Palm	10	39	49	51
Coconut	5	9	14	86

sticks and stones

Even kidney stones seem to be caused by too much fat and carbohydrates in our diet. As Japanese diets have melded into a more Westernized format since World War II, the incidence of calcium oxalate kidney stones has increased. Oxalate, which is found in leafy green vegetables and protein, binds to calcium in urine when the saturation level goes up, due to dehydration or excess excretion of oxalate. Traditionally, stone formers have been told to avoid calcium and foods high in oxalate. But in a study done in Japan, researchers found that carbohydrate consumption and fats were the more likely culprits.[97] Calcium binds to fatty acids in the bowel, indicating that fat consumption may be closely related to oxalate excretion and stone formation. Many types of carbohydrate-rich foods contain a considerable amount of oxalate. High blood sugar increases calcium absorption from the gut in addition to creating higher levels of insulin release.[98] So what's the answer to preventing kidney stones? Eat more protein instead of high glycemic, fat laden carbohydrates.[99]

When it comes to women, the calcium you get from food can prevent kidney stones, while gulping down wads of calcium supplements increases the risk.[100] This is more likely the fault of taking supplements on an empty stomach, when oxalate levels are low, rather than an excess of calcium in the urine. If you're interested in finding more ways to prevent kidney stones, read "The Kidney Stones Handbook" by Gail Savitz and Dr. Stephen Leslie. In another interesting twist, consuming grapefruit juice increased the risk for a kidney stone by 44%, while caffeinated coffee and wine reduced the risk.[101] Grapefruit juice alters the metabolism of many drugs, including estrogen supplements.[102] It seems this particular liquid can alter the breakdown of estrogens through natural flavonoids, making too much 17 beta-estradiol and estrone available to your tissue. So play it on the safe side and take all medication with water.

the protein controversy

Everyone is talking about how dangerous a high protein diet can be, blaming it for everything from osteoporosis to kidney failure. But does it really deserve such a bad rep? Dieticians warn women about too much protein in their diet based upon the recommendations of the American Dietetic Association. However, their conclusions are based upon insulin dependent diabetics and people with compromised vascular problems, especially involving the kidneys. Only recently have dieticians managed the healthy, as most of their work is done in a hospital setting where bodies are under-standably under physical stress.

When women with type 2 diabetes (non-insulin dependent) eat high protein diets, they actually decrease their blood sugar and put less stress on their kidneys than women who eat a low protein, high glycemic carbohydrate diet.[103] Worries about making your body too acid are also unfounded, as sugar and starch cause more acidosis than eating protein.[104] Remember, the more leaky and acidotic a cell becomes, the more rapid premature aging sets in. It seems the arginine in protein actually protects your kidneys' sensitive filtering units.[105] Women suffering from either severe under nutrition, such as anorexia nervosa, or over nutrition have changes in estrogen synthesis and degradation. Studies have suggested that obese women produce more estrogen by using their fat as estrogen converters that simply don't turn off.[106] Anorexic women can't make enough estrogen. By eating protein, you encourage your body to breakdown estrogen quicker which protects sensitive tissue from overexposure to estrogen.

protein kryptonite

By current nutritional standards, eating a diet higher in protein than carbohydrates has received a bad rep in today's press, but a closer look at the mechanisms behind estrogen metabolism may prove it can be your personal kryptonite against cancer caused by too much estrogen in your system. The synthesis and breakdown of estrogen involves enzymes, called cytochrome P-450, in liver and fat cells but also your ovaries. A specific enzyme, estrogen-2-hydroxylase (E2OHase), converts estrone into a non-estrogenic metabolite that is excreted in urine. This enzyme is affected by drugs, body fat and protein in your diet.[107]

the bio-availability of estradiol

By eating protein you encourage your body to breakdown estrogen

The metabolite, 2-OHE, binds to and prevents activation of your estrogen receptors, especially in the uterus. Not so for 16-OHE, which attaches to the same receptor and increases the amount of available circulating estradiol. This can lead to breast cancer and systemic lupus erythematosus, an estrogen-dependent disease.[108,109] Eating a protein rich diet can even increase the activity of your CP-450 enzymes. When individuals were fed a diet composed of 44% protein and 35% carbohydrates, there was a profound affect on the activity in the 2-OHE pathway, favoring estrogen

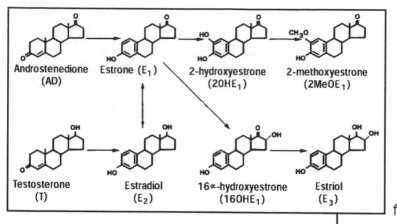

figure 5

deactivation.[110] Even a low fat diet can protect your tissue, shifting estradiol metabolism away from the 16-αhydroxylation pathway and towards the cancer-preventing 2-hydroxylation route.[111] It doesn't take a superwoman to understand that a diet composed of 40% protein, 25% fats and 35% low-glycemic carbohydrates can send you leaping into the air with a single bound!

A diet with 25% fat increases the ability to inactivate estrogen by further shifting the formation of benign, inactive metabolites. It makes sense that high fat diets can contribute to the development of breast and endometrial cancer because they shift the balance towards highly estrogenic, active metabolites.[109,112]

eat like a goddess

Studies of diets emphasizing animal protein are sparse, especially when it comes to understanding how women metabolize protein and fat. When researchers studied the diets of 80,000 women between 34-59 years of age without a previous diagnosis of heart disease, stroke, cancer, diabetes or elevated cholesterol levels, they discovered that replacing carbohydrates with protein was associated with a **lower** risk of heart disease.[113] British researchers concurred, reporting that women who ate the most foods with a low glycemic index – that is, foods that promote a steady, slow rise in blood sugar after a meal, rather than a rapid spike – had high enough levels of the good cholesterol, HDL, and triglycerides to lower their risk of heart disease by 29%.[114]

Scientists still aren't sure how dietary protein affects osteoporosis, even though protein is an important structural component of bone. In a study designed to evaluate the relationship between hip fractures and dietary protein intake, researchers found that eating protein, especially from animal sources, was actually beneficial in reducing the incidence of hip fractures in postmenopausal women followed for ten years.[115] Eating fruits and vegetables high in potassium also protects your bones by reversing any urinary calcium loss.[116] So don't be afraid to eat more protein. It could be just the leg you need to stand on.

friendly phytoestrogens

Phytoestrogens, which are contained in plant foods like garlic and onions, help protect against cancer by pushing the metabolism of estrogen to its less cancerous, inactive metabolites. (Table 7) Phytoestrogens are active in the body and can reduce cholesterol and help treat osteoporosis.[117,118] Garlic and onions seem to offer additional protection against breast cancer while isoflavones, found in beans and soy, had the same effect as hormone replacement therapy on relaxing blood vessels.[119,120]

The source of protein becomes important. Studies have shown protein loading with soybean meal seems to be friendlier on our kidneys than beef or chicken.[121] Some phytoestrogens, like beans and soy, are high in protein. When you enjoy a diet chock-full of these foods, you are really eating a protein adequate diet. So if you are concerned about consuming more protein, just make the difference up with phytoestrogens.[122] Just 40mg of isoflavones per day, the equivalent of one serving of a soy food, equals the typical Asian diet.[123] That's about 3 tablespoons of soy powder or 1.5 ounces of tofu. Just in case you thought eating lots of soy was beneficial, be aware there is a dark side to soy. Too high an intake, especially in supplements, can turn off your

Table 7

---

food sources of phytoestrogens

Isoflavones	<u>Legumes</u> Soy beans, lentils, beans (haricot, broad, kidney, lima, chick peas) <u>Products of beans</u> Soy meal, soy grits, soy flour, tofu, soy milk
Lignans	<u>Whole grain cereals</u> Wheat, wheat germ, barley, hops, rye, rice, brans, oats <u>Fruit, vegetables, seeds</u> Cherries, apples, pears, stone fruits, linseed, sunflower seeds Carrots, fennel, onion, garlic Broccoli Vegetable oils including olive oil <u>Alcoholic sources</u> Beer from hops, bourbon from corn
Coumestans	<u>Bean sprouts</u> Alfalfa, soybean sprouts Fodder crops Clover

---

thyroid and interfere with your hormones, especially estrogen. It's a classic example of soy being beneficial in moderate amounts and harmful in larger amounts, just like estrogen. So use common sense. Incorporate small amounts of low-glycemic phytoestrogens into your diet along with low fat sources of protein for a healthy, goddess lifestyle.

women and alcohol

As someone who grew up in California and makes frequent trips to Napa, I can vouch for the wonderful flavor of California wines. But as a woman, I have to acknowledge wine poses a dangerous risk factor to my health. Unlike men, women who drink alcohol, regardless of the type, increase their chance of getting breast cancer by 12%, making it one of the major avoidable risk factors.[124] Since our stomachs are slower to empty, alcohol has a more intense "first pass" effect on the liver and causes even more delayed emptying.[125] We get higher blood alcohol levels with just one drink. Metabolism of estrogen is intensely affected with blood levels tripling within one hour. Drinking even raises our chances for high blood pressure and strokes.[126-128]

If, like me, you love wine, you should know that women subconsciously crave alcohol as their estrogen levels are dropping. The more we drink the higher estradiol levels can go.[129] But most of all, alcohol makes you fat by increasing your waist and waist-to-hip ratio which correlates with that hidden intra-abdominal fat.[130] In a study comparing the influence of alcohol consumption between French men and women, men had little change in their waist or weight by drinking alcohol, while a woman might as well pour a bottle through her belly button. Women are just more sensitive to the metabolic effects of alcohol and shouldn't be duped into believing the current press that wine is the way to beat heart disease, when a diet rich in fruit and vegetables can provide the same benefits.[131,132,73]

Unfortunately, little effort has been made to provide non-alcoholic wines fortified with quercitin and resveratrol, the active ingredients felt to be responsible for a healthy heart. In the United States, alcohol is the third-leading cause of premature death; its use and abuse result in more than 100,000 deaths annually and imposes more than $167 billion in economic damage on society. The rate of coronary heart disease may be relatively low, but deaths from alcohol-related digestive diseases and cancers, as well as unintentional injuries, are excessive, recently estimated at nearly 25% of all premature mortality. Official government policies in France, as in the United States, call for reductions in alcohol consumption. Does this mean you can't enjoy the occasional glass of Chardonnay? The operative word here is occasional. If you don't want to sabotage

Alcohol makes you fat and raises your chance for high blood pressure and strokes

your shape or increase your risk for certain cancers, keep the wine for that special occasion.

caffeine: grounds for concern?

That cup of joltin' java turns out to be a lot safer than we thought in terms of cancer, but drink too much and you could sabotage your efforts to lose weight by turning off your fat burning mechanism. Dietary caffeine, specifically methylxanthine-containing beverages such as coffee and colas, have been blamed for bone loss, breast cancer and headaches. However, objective studies have been few, relying mostly on supposition and anecdotal experience. But after several studies, caffeine has been given a pardon when it comes to stealing calcium from your bones. One hundred thirty eight postmenopausal women not on estrogen therapy were measured for bone density in their hips and total body. After reviewing their caffeinated beverage use, no incriminating evidence could be found connecting bone loss with caffeine.[133] This was also confirmed in another study where researchers couldn't hang caffeine with causing hip fractures among women who drank regular or decaffeinated coffee, tea or cola.[134] Likewise, over 5000 women with biopsy proven breast cancer were followed for ten years and compared with 5000 women without cancer and no correlation could be found between consumption of caffeine and breast cancer occurrence. In fact, researchers were able to exclude caffeine as a risk factor in breast cancer.[135] And for those of you who can't live without your morning jolt of java, the risk of colon cancer was reduced in drinkers of 4 or more cups per day in over 10,000 people studied for 5 years.[136] However, a rise in blood sugar levels without stimulating insulin was found about 2 hours after drinking caffeine. So if you consume numerous cups a day, you may be turning off glucagon and your fat burning mechanism.[137]

liquid oxygen

Water is an essential but often overlooked nutrient

required for life. Within your body, water is the great transporter of nutrients, oxygen and waste products. It provides a medium for chemical reactions. It cools and cushions your body, which is composed of more than 50% water. In a way, we're a mobile aquarium in which assorted organs slosh around like buoys in an ocean. To be well hydrated the average woman needs to drink 9 cups of fluid per day in the form of nonalcoholic beverages, soups and foods. Solid food contributes about 4 cups of water with an additional 1 cup coming from the process of oxidation in the body. It's been proven that fluid consumption in general and water drinking in particular have a positive effect on the risk of kidney stone disease, breast, colon and urinary tract cancer, obesity, mitral valve prolapse and overall health.[138] Water is really liquid oxygen, made up of two parts hydrogen for every single oxygen molecule. Think of it as just another way of increasing the amount of oxygen in your body. By drinking one liter of mineral water, you can obtain nearly one half of a day's recommended dietary allowance of calcium (1000 milligrams) without any absorption problems. So next time you're reaching for a cola, try some "Liquid Oxygen" instead.

a pinch of salt

We're a mobile aquarium in which organs slosh around like buoys in an ocean

Women have blamed salt for puffy ankles, eyes and those mood changes Al Bundy swore stood for "Pummeling Men's Scrotums"–PMS. But in reality, we need salt to balance our adrenal function. Our bodies are very complex, with the adrenals handling our steroid and salt/water balance. When you become low in salt, your blood pressure drops and you feel light headed. Salt attracts water into our plasma in an effort to compensate for changes in our sympathetic nervous system. While salt sensitivity is an inherited trait in African Americans, it has not been found in other races.[139] When healthy Chinese were given increasing boluses of salt over a week, up to 4250 millimoles a day (that's about 8 tablespoons), there was no change in their blood pressure response.[140] A low salt diet can actually increase your blood glucose and insulin levels, especially if you have any form of hypertension.[141] Afraid salt will make you blow up like a puffer fish in a whistling competition? Not to worry – elevated insulin levels and lower amounts of peripheral deiodination of thyroxine (T4) are to blame.

the thyroid theory

Women with hormone imbalances, and especially postmenopausal women, can develop "subclinical hypothyroidism" detected by the presence of antibodies to the thyroid gland. Nearly 70% of women age 70 have subclinical hypothyroidism which is a risk factor for coronary heart disease.[142] In a study of healthy women, age 35-50, 26% were found to have unsuspected subclinical hypothyroidism identified by the presence of antibodies and higher thyroid stimulating hormone levels than women without antibodies.[143] Yet treatment of this problem with thyroid is controversial and fraught with problems just from the medication alone.[144,145]

Cortisol is necessary to convert T4 into T3 by your thyroid. Women with subclinical hypothyroidism have elevated TSH levels (defined as greater than 2.0) and coincidentally, elevated blood insulin levels or insulin resistance. Remember that insulin will cause you to retain fluid by increasing your sensitivity to salt. Iodine was added to America's salt to prevent mental retardation from thyroid disease caused by iodine-deficient soil in areas such as the Ohio River Valley. However, iodine can cause significant changes in someone who has subclinical hypothyroidism, even in small doses.[146] In Japan seaweed wraps, which come from kelp that is high in iodine, caused marked hypothyroidism among those who ate it daily.[147] So using salt with iodine may be tipping the balance in your thyroid function.

If you taste table salt, it has a bitter flavor due to the chemicals that are added along with the iodine. In comparison, sea salt has a sweet taste. Try switching your salt to a natural sea salt that has not been treated with additional iodine. I bet you will find it takes very little to bring a new flavor balance to your food and your weight.

sweet as sugar

Much has been made about the consumption of sugar in our country, but the intake of fructose has increased steadily in the past two decades as a more natural substitute for sugar in soft drinks and yogurt. However, fructose raises cholesterol and causes more adverse effects on collagen, creating sagging skin and brittle bones.[148] When protein and fructose without any fat or carbohydrate were eaten together, the insulin response was the same as 3 tablespoons of corn syrup. Glucagon was suppressed instead of stimulated in the presence of the combination.[149] So if you plan to eat fruit, either enjoy it one hour before a meal, add some fat or wait at least two hours after having any protein to keep your fat burning metabolism on high.

Aspartame (Nutrasweet™) and other artificial sweeteners have been studied extensively in diabetics.[150] It seems bitter tasting compounds, such as saccharin, sodium cyclamate, stevioside and acesulfame-K stimulate insulin release while sweet tasting aspartame did not.[151] Taste buds are apparently critical in signaling the pancreas to release insulin. Although I could find no studies on sea salt and iodinated salt, I suspect there is a similar response.

the goddess diet

So, you ask, just how does a Goddess diet? The answer is...she doesn't...as a goddess understands how to prevent accelerated metabolic aging by choosing foods that nourish her natural ability to remain fit and strong. But before I summarize everything, I want to be sure you understand that diets don't work...only changes in lifestyle can make a change in your weight. If you don't put yourself at the top of that "TO DO" list, you will let stress and sleeplessness counteract all the good eating habits you'll develop following this program. As you can understand from all I have said in the previous

Fructose raises cholesterol and causes sagging skin

chapters, the regulation of body weight is a deceptively complex process, of which food selection is just one part. Our hormones will fight to hold onto every last globule of fat if we don't gently convince them to get back in line. So how do we accomplish that?

like a trucker's mudflap

If you've ever been behind a big rig on the road, you may have been amused or offended by the figure on a trucker's mudflap. However, if you keep that image in mind, you won't forget the percentage of low glycemic proteins/fats/carbohydrates you should average in a weekly diet:

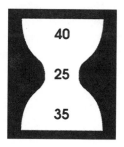

That's right. You want to enjoy 40% of your foods as protein to encourage proper estrogen metabolism; keep your waistline below 30 by selecting 25% of your diet as fats and balance the remaining 35% of your diet with low glycemic carbohydrates to supply your brain with enough glucose for energy. 40/25/35 — that's the plan — and the shape!

You notice I said "average" when giving these percentages. It's unrealistic to think you can manage this ratio at every meal or precisely every day. Dietary intakes vary widely, so it's reasonable to aim for a weekly average. When you eat a meal loaded with more protein, try to make your next meal a little lighter. Remember, by eating small meals frequently, you adjust your insulin response to the next meal which lets you draw or deposit into your carbohydrate savings account, and that spells REFUND when you consciously chose to eat a high glycemic carbohydrate or saturated fat.

How do you know if you are using the recommended "shape" of The Goddess Diet? It's very simple. Just think of your plate as a clock. Fill the portion between 12 and 5 o'clock with protein, the section between 8 and 12 o'clock with low glycemic carbohydrates and the little space left in between nicely holds a mini bowl of fat. As low glycemic carbohydrates contain more fiber, it's impossible to "OD" on them unlike fat, so feel free to use an extra "hour" on that clock.

how many mini meals do I need?

It's very simple to figure out how many mini meals you need. The number of calories you burn at rest is called your basal metabolic rate or BMR. To calculate how many calories you need just to sit still, take your current weight in pounds and multiply by 11. Divide that figure by 250 and you have the number of mini meals necessary just to keep breathing. Now add 250-500 calories for walking, grocery shopping, housework or even just fidgeting and you have an idea of how many calories are required just to maintain your current weight. If you want to lose weight, simply deduct one mini meal and add one half hour of exercise a day to equal an approximate 500 calorie deficit. In just a week you will have lost one pound of fat. Keep it up and you can expect an average weight loss of five pounds the first month, and three pounds each month until you reach your desired goals.

To lose weight, deduct one mini meal and add one half hour of exercise

Don't try to cheat by eliminating two meals and not exercising or eating less than 4 meals a day. You'll just lose muscle and slow down your fat burning metabolism. Then the diet fairy will come visit you and bring back all your fat plus more for good measure. That's a promise.

choosing carbohydrates

Many women prefer to know what they can't eat,

rather than have a long list of all the things allowed on a diet. Since the list of "Don'ts" is rather short, I will get to the point.

Avoid eating these high glycemic carbohydrates until you have achieved a normal BMI.

Apricots	Mango
Baked beans	Muffins
Banana	Noodles
Bread	Oat bran
Carrots	Papaya
Cereals	Parsnips
Corn	Pickles, sweet
Couscous	Potatoes
Cranberry sauce	Raisins
Dates	Rice
Figs	Yams/sweet potatoes

This also means any form of these particular carbohydrates, especially fried or buttered versions, such as potato chips or popcorn. **Remember, high glycemic carbohydrates, when treated with fat, react like 3 tablespoons of corn syrup in your body and prevent you from losing weight.** I don't mean to pronounce a sentence on all these carbohydrates and say you can NEVER eat them again, but if you want to lose the weight and feel more energized, avoid them until you have achieved the following goals:

1. A waistline below 30 inches
2. Body fat percentage below 25%
3. Body mass index below 25

In Chapter 8, I will go over how to calculate your body mass index and fat percentage. It is not weight that determines what is healthy for each of you, but these three factors. If you strive to achieve each one, you will have dropped your risk factors for fat related diseases down to that of a 25 year old goddess. Now that's the true fountain of youth!

find the fat

Your gallbladder needs 10gm of saturated fat at one time in order to empty completely.[152] That is precisely one tablespoon of unsalted butter. Meats and poultry, whether red or white, have varying degrees of saturated fat. Since these are "hidden" fats, that is, you don't see the fat, it is best to restrict your intake of red meat to twice a week. I have found it easiest to restrict my saturated fat by using only 1 tablespoon of unsalted butter a day, and filling the rest of my fat allowance with monounsaturated fats in the form of olive oil. This has the additional advantage of cleaning up your kitchen cupboards, as you no longer need to stock every form of polyunsaturated oil. Extra virgin olive oil contains the highest amount of monounsaturated fatty acids, with the percentage dropping with each subsequent pressing of the olives. However, for salads, I prefer the less flavorful "light" olive oil. Don't confuse the name... there are no differences in calories here, only in the intensity of the flavor.

One tablespoon of butter seems skimpy unless you melt it in a very small container. Pyrex™ produces little glass containers that make a melted tablespoon look enormous. In addition, serving butter this way allows you to dip your low glycemic carbs into it, intensifying the flavor in your mouth while conserving fat grams. And don't forget to grind a few crystals of sea salt into that butter for a sweet, mouth filling flavor.

If you've ever stood in front of the dairy section and worried about choosing the least amount of fat in a product, you may be cheating yourself of a great source for calcium. Research has now shown that calcium binds with fat to form a "soap" which prevents your body from absorbing the fat in cheese and milk.[153] Weight loss in women, especially those with hormone imbalances, improves when you consume more calcium.[154]

California has enriched dairy products with calcium, making 2% milk and cottage cheese the best choice. Kosher yogurt, made with live cultures of acidophilus and no gelatin, offers a whopping 45% of

Variety in your diet is the passbook to your weight savings account

your daily calcium needs in just one cup. Three and one-half ounces of gruyere cheese supplies you with 1011 milligrams of calcium, while cheddar and Monterey Jack provide a respectable 730 milligrams. So don't look at the fat when choosing a dairy product. Read the label and choose the product with the highest percentage of calcium if you're looking to build strong bones AND lose weight. If you find you just crave more saturated fat as you start the diet, try decreasing the frequency instead of the amount of saturated fat you eat in a day. Again, the French have proven variety in your diet is the passbook to your weight savings account.

protecting with protein

There are several reasons to eat more protein than currently recommended, especially in light of its ability to direct estrogen metabolism. But too much protein can stress kidneys already affected by atherosclerotic disease. The current recommendations are to consume no more than 15-20% of your diet as protein. As I have already discussed, soy protein does not cause super filtration in the kidney and provides our bodies with numerous benefits in fighting cancer and regulating cholesterol. By adding an additional 15% protein in the form of soy, you can improve your cholesterol and help protect your breast and uterine lining from any stimulation by estrogen. This is a GREAT thing!

It's easy to add soy to your diet with all the products available in today's supermarket. Try adding a tofu dog to a cup of soup, or sprinkle the powder into a hot bowl of Irish oatmeal. It's a natural for stir fry and blends up easily with Swiss Miss™ Diet Chocolate drink. Eat it as cheese or drink soy milk. The possibilities are endless. Learning to cook with soy can benefit your entire family. If you come up with a creative way to utilize soy in your diet, share it with others by posting it on my website at **http://www.goddessdiet.com**. You'll find other helpful hints and medical information, motivational audio tapes, a newsletter, products of interest to women and a message board so you can share your struggles and success. So join in with others in making The Goddess

Diet your healthy lifestyle.

fruit smoothies and energy bars

It's tempting to suggest you have a fruit smoothie for breakfast and they have become a popular way to get energy on the run. However, when protein and fructose, the natural sugar in fruit, are combined without any fat, the response in the body is the same as if you ate several pieces of white bread or swallowed 3 tablespoons of corn syrup. So don't make the mistake of mixing a protein powder, such as whey or soy with water and fruit. Always make a protein drink with 2% milk. You'll keep your insulin and glucose levels under control and still have a tasty, nutritious treat. A liquid breakfast, however, doesn't balance your insulin response as well as a high fiber meal because it is absorbed at a much faster rate.[155] It's okay to use a liquid breakfast once a week, but don't make a habit of it or you'll find yourself hunting for those dangerous high sugar carbs before lunch.

When choosing fruits for your diet, concentrate on red/purple or dark blue fruits such as blueberries, blackberries, plums, huckleberries or dark red ones such as raspberries. Not only are they lower in fructose but they contain proanthocyanidins (PCA's) which can strengthen blood vessels such as capillaries and help to prevent wrinkles, varicose veins or bruising. When choosing grapefruit, red fruit contains more vitamins than pale yellow fruit with almost three times as much Vitamin A and C.

Energy bars are another area of potential danger. Composed of protein and carbohydrates, these bars use fructose, rice, barley or corn syrup as a sweetener and can create a "Buddha Belly" faster than you can chant a mantra! Look for new protein bars by MetRx called "Source One" which are low in fructose, sucrose and fat. As more nutrition companies focus on helping women control their glucose response, you can bet we'll see more products coming down the pipeline.

eat like an elephant

Putting away a few nuts may help you lose weight and protect your heart. Peanuts, almonds, macadamia, walnuts and cashews are excellent sources of monounsaturated fats which can keep your arteries clean as a whistle. These calorie-dense snacks are versatile and easy to incorporate into meals. Just 5 ounces is enough to provide you with 50% of your daily Vitamin E and folic acid requirements, which lowers your risk of heart disease. Nuts also contain resveratrol, the compound in red wine that prevents the oxidation of LDL in your blood. Nuts won't add inches to your waistline if eaten in small quantities but they will go a long way in helping you feel satisfied with less saturated fat in your diet. Dry roasted, unsalted peanuts are ideal for snacking and cooking. A handful is about 2 ounces, so go ahead...toss them in a salad or stew. Just don't forget to use them.

Nuts may help you lose weight and protect your heart

the spice in life

There is nothing more likely to evoke memories of home cooking than the smell of spices. Having traveled most of the "free inoculum world" or anyplace where you don't need a vaccination, I can instantly recall a country by its smell. Cardamom, anise and cloves in Denmark to cumin, cinnamon and turmeric in Morocco—each of these combinations gets my digestive juices flowing. Herbs de Provence, a combination of french lavender, basil, thyme, savory and fennel gives all foods a new zip. As an additional benefit, fennel seeds (also known as fenugreek) help to lower blood glucose.[156] Don't forget that salt is a spice. Sometimes just a few grinds of sea salt followed by a great cracked pepper is all you need to make a gourmet dinner. Experiment with the numerous spice combinations available commercially in your market. In Appendix A of this book and on my website I will give you places to order exotic and unusual spices. With just a little variety you can make cooking as adventuresome as a trip around the world.

tea time

Tea is a medicinal drink in many cultures and a sign of friendship, as in Middle Eastern countries. Who isn't aware of the British penchant for afternoon tea or the symbolism of dumping it into Boston Harbor? Teas are really an infusion of hot water into the leaf of a plant in order to extract its essence. Some teas, such as green tea have compounds felt to protect against cancer. One cup of green or black tea has more antioxidant power than one-half cup of broccoli, carrots, spinach or stawberries. Just by drinking two cups a day, women can lower their risk of aortic atherosclerosis by 46%, and when you drink 4 cups the risk drops by 69%.[157] With the wide variety of teas available, it's fun to make a different flavor every day. Mango and papaya teas contain enzymes that can help with your digestion of fats and proteins. It can be made by either placing a jar of cold water in the sun to process, called sun tea, leaving it out overnight, called moon tea or by infusing the mixture with hot water for 5 minutes. Look for decaffeinated teas whenever possible as they are less acidic. I enjoy Tejava, a mineral water tea made by Crystal Geyser Water Company which is available in your grocery store.

the hidden sugar: corn syrup

I was amazed when I seriously began to study food labels and discovered how many products contain corn syrup. Sold as glucose in England, corn syrup is in everything from tomato soup and juice to coffee cream substitutes. Due to the enormous excess of corn production in this country, it has become the number one sweetener in commercial products. And don't fall for rice or barley syrup as a substitute. They all have the same effect in your body. High fructose corn syrup depletes your body of vitamins and minerals and can lead to intracellular dehydration and aging. It's critical that you read the entire label on any product as you could inadvertently send your weight management program barreling off track by a simple mistake, leaving you to wonder how those fat pads hitched a ride on your hips. But here's an interesting thought—if you stick to the fresh produce section instead of the aisles of the supermarket, you won't have to be so diligent.

msg by so many names

Steering clear of monosodium glutamate, or MSG, is about as easy as dodging death or taxes. Twenty million Americans are estimated to be sensitive to this food additive which is required by the FDA to be listed whenever it is an ingredient in foods. However, there is no law requiring manufacturers to declare components of any ingredient. Additives such as hydrolyzed vegetable protein (HVP), autolyzed yeast or yeast extract, and sodium and calcium caseinate all contain potentially threatening amounts of MSG, making up between 8 to 40 percent of HVP. Again, as it is used mainly as a preservative and flavor enhancing agent, that's another good reason to stay in the produce section.

portions: do they matter?

The issue of portion control is a hot one in weight management. If you're hungry, you will eat bigger portions because your brain doesn't get the signal from your stomach that it's full and had enough. Remember, hormones in your gut are responsible for emailing your brain to tell your hand to put the fork down. The greatest reason for lack of portion control is the hormonal imbalance created by delayed gastric emptying.

When I gained my weight, I was accused of having a "wooden leg" because I could eat large portions of food without feeling full. Convinced this was a misperception, I bought a kitchen scale and weighed out a single recommended portion of protein – 3 oz. It was disgustingly scrawny! I couldn't possibly exist on that little protein for my one, big meal of the day. Then I measured out a dry serving of pasta – 2 oz. My birds eat more noodles than that! Although I never tallied my calorie consumption, it was clear I was eating for more than one.

I started on The Goddess Diet without any concern for portion control and an interesting thing happened. I began cooking from the refrigerator and not the cupboard. When I started nibbling on protein first, I discovered my eyes were indeed bigger than my stomach. I stopped skipping breakfast and started to eat 5 or more meals a day. Within a week I was no longer hungry and I didn't miss the high glycemic carbohydrates I had made a staple in my diet. I was letting my body send the proper hormonal signals through cholecystokinin and glucagon to my brain. I was actually leaving food on my plate for the first time.

But things got even better. I began saving time and money when I shopped. By starting at the fresh produce and dairy sections, I had little need for trips down the aisles filled with shelf-stable high glycemic carbohydrates or a stop at the bakery. I experimented with the wide range of available fresh fish and selected only lean red meat for my twice weekly indulgence. The amount of food I bought dropped as I realized I could do with smaller portions of meat and more vegetables and fruit. I can now tell you, five years later, I cut my grocery bill in half by using the principles in The Goddess Diet. And who can't use more time or money? Remember, each bite of food gives you a new opportunity to revitalize and energize your metabolism, so choose wisely!

principles of the goddess diet

Consume a diet averaging:

- 40% protein to encourage proper estrogen metabolism

- 25% fat (15% monounsaturated fats and 10% saturated)

- 35% low glycemic carbohydrates

- Eat 5 mini meals a day beginning with breakfast

- Exercise 30 minutes a day

- Eat 1 serving of soy a day

- Begin every meal with a mini protein starter

- Use non-iodinated sea salt

- Enjoy 5 ounces of nuts a week

- Avoid alcoholic beverages

- Drink 4 eight ounce glasses of water a day, preferably mineral water

- Reduce caffeine

- Eat low fat but not non-fat dairy products

- Use 1 tablespoon of unsalted butter daily

- Never consume fruit and proteins together without fat

- If you eat a high glycemic carbohydrate, don't add fat

chapter four

cooking with a food surgeon

I was not "born to cook". Even my genes were against it. Though my mother was raised on a wheat farm in Assiniboia, Saskatchewan, Canada, she could present a turkey so undercooked I felt obligated to resuscitate it. They say some things skip generations, but whatever chromosome the cooking gene is on, it seems to have skipped a lot more than that in my family.

As a child raised in the San Fernando Valley, the only taste of decent cooking I ever had was when my grandmother would come to visit for the winter. I eagerly waited for her to bring out preserves she carefully brought down on the train, introducing me to goose-berries and red currants in exotic, quilted jars that glistened in the sunlight on the porch, where they were stored for those special occasions that never came. We actually ate something other than porridge for breakfast during her visits and I was in awe that scrambled eggs didn't have to contain the shells in order to provide a complete, nutritious meal. Let's face it—my mother burned water which is why I was ten before I learned the fire alarm wasn't a kitchen timer.

Dinner at home was more like attending a lynching than a family gathering. No one could decide upon a proper topic of conversation so everyone just shouted for as long as it took to divide up the spoils of the evening that were placed before them. Then silence would descend as we tried to identify parts even another chicken couldn't recognize. Some nights I prayed the oven could flush.

It's no wonder that, after suffering from a medical scare at the tender age of 5 that led me to believe I might only live a few years, I quietly told my parents I wanted to be a doctor. It was that simple. Now, 45 years later, I think of myself as a "Food Surgeon", dissecting nutrition labels instead of bodies, patching up recipes so they can fulfill their destiny – to help each of us live a healthy life. Even my kitchen, with all my knives in graduated, sharpened order, could sub as an operating room in the event of a disaster if it weren't for the floating dog hair and bird seed scattered on the floor. So let me share with you "secrets" to making food your home pharmacy.

sweet talk

Sugar and spice make everything nice, especially when you use seasonings that contain chromium, a nutrient that helps to maintain insulin sensitivity in your tissues. Scientists have discovered that spices such as cinnamon, tumeric, cloves, bay leaves and fennel seeds can triple insulin's ability to sweep glucose into your hungry cells.[158] No wonder Greek, Mexican and the nomadic cultures of North Africa favor these spices in their cooking. You will find the recipes in this chapter make extensive use of these flavor accents. And don't be afraid to add a little sugar to any of the recipes. Although I have designed the 250 calorie mini meals without the addition of sugar, research has shown that sugar, when added to foods, has no additional effect on blood glucose levels than those of the sugar alone, and can prevent you from increasing your intake of fat and high glycemic carbohydrates.[159]

salt: the new luxury ingredient

It's reported in the Bible that God turned Lot's wife into a pillar of salt when she disobeyed His instructions not to look back at the destruction of Sodom and Gomorrah. Fortunately, I can promise you no such disaster will befall you if you indulge in the new luxury ingredient of the millennium – natural sea salt. For several decades, salt has been blamed for a host of diseases, but suddenly, it's coming back into favor. Salt

Spices such as cinnamon, tumeric, cloves, bay leaves and fennel seeds can triple insulin's ability to sweep glucose into your hungry cells

is every bit as essential to our health and survival as when we first shed those flippers and scales and emerged from the sea and migrated inland.

Salt wakes up the flavor in food and improves the taste of almost everything, allowing flavors to mature and come into harmony in a dish. Today you can purchase a selection of sea salts that can sparkle like the crown jewels when you scatter them over summer-ripe tomatoes or grind a few crystals over fish or pork.

it's an egg-xaggeration

The egg may not be the cholesterol-raising culprit it was once believed, especially if you are already eating a low-saturated fat diet. It seems diets high in carbohydrates impair your glucose tolerance and increase your triglyceride levels while reducing the good cholesterol in NIDDM individuals.[160] In fact, researchers are rethinking cholesterol's role in cardiovascular crimes. It seems people vary widely in their ability to metabolize cholesterol, and compensate for absorbed dietary cholesterol by decreasing the amount produced in the liver or by increasing the cholesterol excreted, along with bile, from the gallbladder. Even eating 21 eggs a week can't make cholesterol stick around in healthy, young women.[161] And if you want to protect your eyes, nothing can beat the humble egg yolk as the nutritional champ for levels of the carotenoids, lutein and zeaxanthin.[162] So try the omelette recipes in the book and remember – if the cholesterol don't stick...you must acquit!

the chocolate diet

No, I'm not recommending your consume a diet based on chocolate, but including some in your weekly Goddess Diet Plan won't cause any harm. It seems cocoa butter contains stearic acid, which can actually drop your cholesterol levels.[163] Although it is a highly saturated fat, it's melting point is above body temperature, making it less well absorbed. I myself am partial to a California product by Scharffen Berger that contains 70% cocoa butter, but in a pinch I have been known to munch on a Dove silky dark chocolate chunk or a Snickers bar, all of which have been tested and found to fall in the moderate range for raising your blood sugar levels.[164] If you want to see the full listing of foods tested to date, and their GI ratings, read "The Glucose Revolution: The Authoritative Guide to the Glycemic Index" by Miller and Wolever or connect to http://www.mendosa.com/gi.htm on the web. This site contains a wealth of information about the GI values of food and is constantly updated as new research becomes available.

the non-nutrient: fiber

Increasing fiber in your diet can help protect sensitive tissues from too long an exposure to active estrogens such as estrone and estradiol. It seems having a regular bowel movement reduces the time estrogens have to be reabsorbed from stool in the colon, which cuts down on the amount of circulating estrogen.[165] It can also keep your blood sugar in check while helping with weight loss. Women should focus on including as many fiber-rich foods in their diet, especially pears, apples and beans. I have included several recipes that make sure you obtain enough insoluble fiber to keep those hemorrhoids that were a gift from your childbearing years in seclusion.

the stinking rose

Garlic and members of the onion family, such as leeks, shallots, chives and scallions, have been used to treat an array of ills since the dawn of civilization. Packed full of antioxidants, these foods can help protect against cancer, elevated cholesterol levels and strokes. They were even used to protect against food poisoning by the ancient Mesopotamians. I have used them liberally throughout The Goddess Diet not only for their flavor, but to demonstrate how easy it is to make food your own personal healer.

the goddess diet mini meal menu plan

Let's look at a sample 7-day menu plan for someone who needs to eat 5 meals a day, or 1250 calories. If you use the ratios of The Goddess Diet, you would need to eat the following amounts of protein/fat/carbs:

Calories	Protein 40%	Fat 25%	Sat 10%	Carbs 35%
1250	500	312.5	125	437.5
1500	600	375	150	525
1750	700	437	175	612
2000	800	500	200	700

Now look at the number of grams that represents, remembering that 1 gram equals 9 fat calories but only 4 calories from protein or carbohydrates.

Calories	Protein GM	Fat GM	Sat GM	Carbs GM
1250	125	34.7	14	109.3
1500	150	41	16	131
1750	175	48.6	19	153.4
2000	200	55	22	175

day 1

Meal	*Calories*
1. Connemara Irish oatmeal (p. 110)	304
2. Tuna and white bean salad (p. 75)	275
3. Calcutta chicken in spinach and yogurt sauce (p. 92)	235
Winter fruit salad (p. 116)	76
4. Fourth of July cottage cheese (p.136)	227
5. Seared black scallops (p. 85)	138
Chilled cantaloupe and mint soup (p. 77)	104

Total
Cal: 1362
Protein: 130 g
Carbs: 136 g
Fat: 37 g
Sat: 10 g

day 2

1. Bahian black bean chili (p.112)	221
2. Fourth of July cottage cheese (p. 136)	227
3. Cuban grilled skirt steak (p. 99)	159
Leeks Nicoise (p. 101)	109
4. Grilled chicken and mandarin orange salad (p. 74)	273
5. Tu Tu Tun grilled lodge salmon (p. 90)	250
Kabocha squash with Tunisian flavors (p. 104)	50

Total
Cal: 1291
Protein: 125 g
Carbs: 121 g
Fat: 39 g
Sat: 11 g

day 3

1. Provencal style lemon sole (p. 88)	210
2. Carlos and Charlie's tuna dip (p. 133)	69
Thai shrimp broth with lemongrass, chili and ginger (p.82)	121
3. Mussels in chipotle chile broth (p. 86)	178
Moroccan orange salad (p. 71)	70
4. Baked Basque cod (p. 91)	140
Aztec zucchini (p. 102)	95
5. Indian turkey cutlets (p. 96)	154
Red lentil and tofu curry (p. 113)	137

Total
Cal: 1201
Protein: 133 g
Carbs: 78 g
Fat: 38 g
Sat: 7 g

day 4

Meal	Calories
1. Rogue River salmon omelette (p. 65)	186
Joel's asparagus bake (p. 108)	32
2. Crab with spicy orange dressing (p.69)	138
Yogurt and nuts (p. 134)	161
3. Lemon tarragon chicken (p. 94)	223
Zucchini noodles with spicy tomato sauce (p. 106)	44
4. Strawberries with cassis, balsamic vinegar and mint (p. 116)	180
5. Sea bass with chili and saffron (p. 86)	261

Total
Cal: 1225
Protein: 119 g
Carbs: 106 g
Fat: 39 g
Sat: 11 g

day 5

Meal	Calories
1. Fennel and lemon soup (p. 80)	150
Spiced fruit salad (p. 118)	107
2. Shrimp salad (p. 72)	274
3. Moorish spicy lamb kebabs (p. 97)	165
Rosemary and lemon pinto beans (p. 111)	96
4. Chicken, tofu and watercress stir-fry (p. 93)	159
Stir-fried bok choy (p. 105)	86
5. Herbed tomato juice (p. 137)	37
Halibut with artichokes, zucchini, tomatoes (p. 85)	208
Tuscany eggplant (p. 134)	57

Total
Cal: 1340
Protein: 133 g
Carbs: 110 g
Fat: 45 g
Sat: 8 g

day 6

Meal	Calories
1. Rogue River salmon omelette (p. 65)	186
Smoky "virgin" mary (p. 138)	26
2. Cream of bell pepper soup (p. 79)	94
Shrimp with two mushrooms (p. 88)	165
3. Roasted turkey breast (p. 93)	70
Apple, walnut, grapes and celery salad (p. 73)	162
Sassy rhubarb mint coolers (p. 138)	19
4. Sear-roasted halibut (p.89)	183
Tomato and caper sauce (p. 125)	54
5. Pork chops with chipotle marinade (p. 100)	175
Roasted peaches with cardamom (p. 114)	78

Total
Cal: 1216
Protein: 133 g
Carbs: 74 g
Fat: 45 g
Sat: 12 g

day 7

Meal	Calories
1. Breakfast protein shake	192
2. Tomato and pumpkin soup (p. 80)	110
Garbanzos with garlic and kale (p.109)	122
3. Spicy beef with basil (p. 98)	217
Yellow tomato, watermelon, arugula salad (p. 117)	96
4. Grilled eggplant dip (p. 134)	123
Veggies for dip	54
5. Orange roughy with orange, caper and olive sauce (p. 83)	190
Balsamic roasted squash and apples (p.103)	109

Total
Cal: 1217
Protein: 92 g
Carbs: 138 g
Fat: 39 g
Sat: 7 g

weekly average

Cal: 1261
Protein: 124 g (38%)
Carbs: 109 g (34%)
Fat: 40 g (28%)
Sat: 9 g (7%)

As you can see, it's all just a balancing act when you're trying to lose weight, so don't be afraid to put a little "wiggle" into your diet. It's what you take in over several days that counts, not each and every bite. Even the overweight steelworker in "The Full Monty" recognized "the less I eat...the fatter I get!" So do like his friend advised...just "stuff yourself and get thin" with The Goddess Diet Plan.

I recognize we, as goddesses, have no time to waste in the kitchen when there is so much life to experience, so I have designed The Goddess Diet Mini Meals to be quick and delicious. I promise you won't need a certificate from a cooking school to understand the recipes. In a way, you could say The Goddess Diet is not about changing your life, but rather having the time of your life making choices that can only lead to a healthier, more youthful you!

eggs

basil pistou omelette

Serves 8
per portion
Calories: 94
Protein: 8 g
Carbs: 1 g
Fat: 6 g
Sat: 2 g

Pistou is the French version of Italian pesto, only the pine nuts are missing. Here I have used it to make a wonderful flavoring for a large omelette. Use only fresh basil leaves for the best flavor.

3 garlic cloves, chopped
1 cup fresh basil leaves, washed and dried
sea salt, white pepper
1 tablespoon extra-virgin olive oil
1/2 cup grated Parmesan cheese
4 eggs and 4 egg whites
1 tablespoon water

Put the garlic, basil, salt, pepper and 1 tablespoon oil in a food processor and blend until smooth. Add the cheese, a little at a time, until a very stiff paste forms. Set aside.

Whisk the eggs with salt, pepper and water until foamy. Spray a mist of olive oil on a large, nonstick omelette pan and heat until it is very hot. Add the egg mixture and let it cook 5 seconds. As the eggs begin to set, lift the edge with a fork and tilt the pan to run the eggs underneath. Continue until almost set but still slightly soft inside, about 30 seconds. Remove from the heat.

Quickly spread the pistou over the eggs and fold the omelette onto a serving plate to form a slight roll. Serve immediately.

allah's sunrise

This recipe comes from the Middle East and can be made as spicy as you or your family can tolerate. I enjoyed it one morning as the sun was rising over the Great Atlas Mountains in Morocco. The owner of the little store on the route to Marrakech let me watch him prepare this regional dish while his goat nibbled on the few bunches of grass outside the door.

Serves 2
per portion
Calories: 197
Protein: 9 g
Carbs: 19 g
Fat: 10 g
Sat: 2.6 g

2 teaspoons extra virgin olive oil
1/3 cup chopped white onion
1/2 green bell pepper, seeded and cut into strips
1/2 poblano or red bell pepper,
    seeded and cut into strips
1 jalapeno pepper, raw, seeded and cut into tiny strips
    (retain the seeds and add for additional hotness)
8 ounces Muir Glen organic crushed tomatoes
    (see Resources)
2 teaspoons cayenne pepper or Aleppo pepper
    (see Resources)
sea salt
2 large eggs
Freshly ground black pepper to taste

Heat an empty cast iron skillet dry on medium heat, then add the olive oil and saute the onions and sweet peppers until soft, about 5 minutes, stirring with a wooden spoon.

Add the jalapeno and tomatoes and cook until the mixture just begins to thicken, about 8 minutes. Add the Aleppo or cayenne pepper and some sea salt to taste and adjust the seasoning for your preference.

Break one egg at a time into a bowl and slide it into the skillet while the tomato and pepper mixture is simmering. Cook for another 8 minutes, spooning the sauce over the eggs until they are set. Divide the dish in half and serve in individual bowls topped with black pepper.

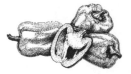

rogue river salmon omelette

Serves 2
per portion
Calories: 186
Protein: 20 g
Carbs: 5 g
Fat: 9 g
Sat: 3 g

Fishing on the Rogue River in Oregon is one of the simple delights in life. Chinook, Steelhead and Coho salmon run the river year round creating quite a boat traffic jam during high season. This delicious omelette is a fragrant reminder of the bounties of nature.

1 large egg and 3 egg whites
sea salt
pepper
3 ounces smoked salmon
1 ounce goat cheese
4 small cherry tomatoes, split in half
2 tablespoons fresh parsley

Preheat oven to 350 degrees. In a small electric mixing bowl, beat egg whites with salt and pepper till stiff peaks form. In another bowl, lightly beat yolks with a fork. Fold whites into yolks.

Lightly grease an oven proof nonstick skillet and place over medium-high heat. Spread the egg mixture in the pan. Cook 3 to 5 minutes or until the bottom is lightly golden.

Place skillet in the hot oven on a medium rack and bake for 3 minutes or until nearly dry.

Dot with the goat cheese, salmon, tomatoes and parsley and bake 1 minute more. To serve, fold the omelette in half.

french feta and zucchini frittata

Serves 4
per portion
Calories: 175
Protein: 11 g
Carbs: 3 g
Fat: 13 g
Sat: 6 g

This is a rich dish, but well worth splurging some fat calories on for a special breakfast.

3 large eggs plus 4 egg whites
1/2 cup half-and-half
2 teaspoons extra-virgin olive oil
1 cup zucchini noodles (p.106)
2 ounces fresh French feta cheese
1 teaspoon chopped dill

Preheat the broiler. In a a large bowl beat the eggs with the half-and-half and season lightly with salt and pepper.

In a heavy 9-inch oven-proof skillet, warm the olive oil over moderately high heat. When the oil begins to shimmer, add the eggs. Reduce the heat to moderately low and scatter the zucchini noodles over the eggs. Dot with the cheese and sprinkle with the dill. Cover and cook until almost set, about 12 minutes.

Broil the frittata for about 2 minutes or until the eggs are set. Cut into wedges and serve.

classic french omelette

The first thing I was taught at cooking school in France was how to make an omelette. I've adapted this recipe to include soy and my favorite herbs de Provence.

1 teaspoon extra-virgin olive oil
1/2 cup zucchini, diced
2 green onions, sliced
1 large egg and 3 egg whites
3 teaspoons soy powder
1/2 cup water
1/4 teaspoon herbs de Provence (see Resources)
sea salt

Serves 2
per portion
Calories: 139
Protein: 16 g
Carbs: 7 g
Fat: 5 g
Sat: 1 g

In a small nonstick skillet saute the zucchini and green onions over medium heat until soft.

In a separate bowl beat the eggs and egg white with the soy powder and add enough water for consistency. Pour the mixture over the vegetables and season with salt and herbs de Provence. Split the cherry tomatoes in half and place on the left side of the omelette. When the mixture is nearly set, slide the omelette onto a plate, tipping the pan to fold the omelette in half.

salads

cucumber-yogurt salad

Serves 6
per portion
Calories: 70
Protein: 3 g
Carbs: 5 g
Fat: 4 g
Sat: 2 g

This cooling salad has many names in the eastern and Mediterranean culture and even appears in Egypt and the Middle East. To make the best tasting salad, drain the yogurt for 2 hours before mixing.

2 cups whole milk yogurt
sea salt
1/2 medium cucumber, peeled and seeded
3 to 4 garlic cloves, mashed in a mortar and pestle
1 tablespoon chopped fresh dill
2 teaspoons fresh mint
2 teaspoons extra-virgin olive oil
1 tablespoon lemon juice

Combine the yogurt and 1/4 teaspoon sea salt in a cheesecloth-lined strainer over a bowl and let it drain for 2 hours.

Grate the cucumber with a coarse grater to make 1 cup total. Place the grated cucumber in another cheesecloth-lined strainer. Salt lightly and let drain 30 minutes.

Combine the yogurt, cucumber, garlic, herbs and olive oil. Mix well. Add the lemon juice to taste and season with salt. Let sit 1 hour before using.

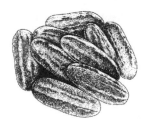

grilled steak and asparagus salad

This makes a wonderful, quick meal on a hot, summer day. Serve it with a garden-fresh salad for a meal even your friends will envy.

Serves 6
per portion
Calories: 162
Protein: 20 g
Carbs: 3 g
Fat: 8 g
Sat: 2 g

Vinaigrette:
1/4 cup hoisin sauce
1/4 cup white wine vinegar
1/4 cup canned fat free, reduced sodium chicken broth
4 teaspoons extra-virgin olive oil
4 teaspoons minced peeled fresh ginger
1 tablespoon soy sauce
2 teaspoons hot Chinese-style mustard or Dijon mustard

Salad:
1 tablespoon black peppercorns
2 teaspoons coriander seeds
2 teaspoons fennel seeds
1 1-pound top sirloin steak (about 1 inch thick)
Olive oil spray
1 pound thin asparagus spears, trimmed
3 medium-thin red onion slices
Orange slices

For vinaigrette: Blend all ingredients in a blender until smooth. Season with sea salt and pepper.

For salad: Grind peppercorns, coriander seeds and fennel seeds to a fine powder. Lightly spray steak with olive oil and sprinkle each side with salt, pepper and 1-1/2 teaspoons spice mix. Let stand 30 minutes.

Prepare barbecue (medium-high heat). Grill steak until cooked to desired doneness, about 5 minutes per side for medium-rare. Using tongs so as not to pierce the meat, transfer steak to a cutting board and let rest for 10 minutes, covered with foil.

While the steak is taking a much needed rest, (but not you!) spray the asparagus and onion slices with olive oil and sprinkle with salt and pepper. Grill asparagus until crisp-tender and slightly charred, turning often, about 5 minutes. Transfer to a plate and repeat with onion slices, keeping them intact.

Cut steak crosswise into thin slices. Arrange steak and asparagus on 6 plates. Drizzle with vinaigrette and garnish with onion rings and orange slices.

crab with spicy orange dressing

Serves 6
per portion
Calories: 138
Protein: 13 g
Carbs: 10 g
Fat: 5 g
Sat: 2 g

This dressing is excellent on shrimp, scallops or lobster and makes the fennel unusually sweet. Try using grapefruit juice instead of orange for another tasty variation. I have even served sections of grapefruit with this salad.

1 medium bulb fennel
1 tablespoon extra-virgin olive oil
3 tablespoons lemon juice
sea salt, pepper
2 cups fresh squeezed orange juice (grapefruit or lime)
1 teaspoon ancho chili powder (see Resources)
1 tablespoon unsalted butter
3 cans fancy white crab meat, picked for shells
1 1/2 tablespoons ground cumin
1/4 teaspoon cayenne pepper
8 basil leaves

Trim the top and bottom of the fennel bulb, then quarter lengthwise and slice the quarters into 1/8 inch slices. Place in a mixing bowl and toss with the olive oil, 2 tablespoons lemon juice and season to taste with salt and pepper.

In a small saucepan, bring the orange juice, remaining lemon juice and chili powder to a simmer over medium-high heat. Reduce to 1/3 cup, 15-17 minutes. Remove from the heat and whisk in the butter.

Drain the crab and check for any shell fragments. Mix with the ground cumin and cayenne pepper.

To serve, mound the fennel strips on the plate, press down in the middle and arrange the crab meat mixture on top. Drizzle the reduced orange dressing around the base of the fennel and over the crab.

Stack basil leaves and cut in julienne strips. Sprinkle on top of the crab.

lemon chicken

This version of chicken is full of lemon flavor and bite. I use lemons preserved Morrocan style to add an exotic taste to this dish. Try freezing the chicken so it is easier to slice thinly.

1 1/4 pound skinless, boneless chicken breast halves,
    partially frozen
1 tablespoon canola oil
2 cups dry white wine
Juice of lemon
sea salt, pepper
1 bunch watercress, stems discarded
1 large head radicchio leaves, separated
2 preserved lemons,
    thinly sliced crosswise for garnish*

Serves 6
per portion
Calories: 170
Protein: 13 g
Carbs: 1 g
Fat: 3 g
Sat: <1 g

Using a sharp knife, thinly slice each chicken breast half on the diagonal 1/2 inch thick. Pound the chicken slices in a plastic bag until they are 1/4 inch thick.

Heat a large skillet on medium high heat dry, then add 1 tablespoon oil and half the chicken and cook until barely done, about 1 minutes per side; it will still be opaque in places. Transfer the chicken to a plate and repeat with the rest of the chicken, adding oil as necessary.

Carefully add the wine and lemon juice to the skillet, season with salt and pepper and bring to a boil over high heat. Return the chicken to the skillet and cook, stirring constantly, until the slices are white, about 2 to 3 minutes.

Line a platter with the watercress and radicchio and arrange the chicken slices on top. Garnish with the preserved lemon slices and serve immediately.

* To preserve lemons, rinse and scrub lemons or limes to remove any wax. Cut each fruit almost into four pieces by making cuts at right angles to each other from one end of the fruit almost to the other, leaving enough fruit uncut so that the lemon can be opened without falling apart, about 1/2 inch. Generously salt the exposed flesh with sea salt, using at least 3 tablespoons per pound of fruit. Put the salted fruits in a big, clean jar and cover

with fresh lemon juice or water. Lemon juice gives a better flavor, but don't use bottled lemon juice. Put on the lid and leave the jar at room temperature for four or five weeks.

moroccan orange salad

Serves 4
per portion
Calories: 70
Protein: 1 g
Carbs: 10 g
Fat: 4 g
Sat: <1 g

This salad was served to me in Agadir, Morocco where the evening ocean breeze is filled with the fragrance of roses. You can make this salad with either daikon (a large white radish) or fennel. One taste and your guests will be looking for your magic lamp, so make plenty.

2 small oranges
1 daikon
mint springs

Dressing:
1 tablespoon lemon juice
2 teaspoons orange-flower water (see Resources)
1 tablespoon extra-virgin olive oil
sea salt, pepper
1 tablespoon chopped mint

Peel the oranges, removing the pith and slice. Peel the daikon and slice in thin circles. Arrange the daikon and oranges in an alternating pattern on a dish.

Make the dressing by whisking together lemon juice, orange-flower water, olive oil, salt and pepper. Pour dressing over the slices and sprinkle with the chopped mint and refrigerate.

Garnish with mint sprigs and serve.

shrimp salad

Here's an example of soyamaise at work with shrimp.

1 pound extra-large shrimp, peeled and deveined
2 tablespoons lemon juice
sea salt, white pepper
One bag of romaine lettuce or 2 large heads
6 tablespoons soyamaise (recipe on p. 132)

Serves 4
per portion
Calories: 183
Protein: 28 g
Carbs: 5 g
Fat: 6 g
Sat: 0 g

Marinate the shrimp in the lemon juice. Season with salt and pepper, then place under the broiler or on the grill, cooking them until uniformly pink and firm, about 2 minutes per side.

Assemble the salad in individual serving bowls. Tear the lettuce into pieces and toss with the soyamaise.

Add the shrimp and serve.

apple, walnut, grapes and celery salad

Serves 2
per portion
Calories: 108
Protein: 1 g
Carbs: 16 g
Fat: 5 g
Sat: 1 g

Poor Mr. Fawlty got a lesson in making a Waldorf salad when a rude, American guest stayed at his establishment. I promise you this salad will make no demands.

2 tablespoons reduced fat mayonnaise
1 tablespoon fresh lemon juice
1 crisp red apple
2 tablespoons walnuts
1/3 cup grapes
1-1/2 celery stalks
sea salt, pepper

In a non-metallic bowl, whisk together the mayonnaise and lemon juice, salt and pepper to taste until combined.

Cut celery and apple into 1-1/2-inch long thin julienne strips. Toss together the apple, walnuts, grapes and celery with the dressing.

strawberries and feta salad

Serves 4
per portion
Calories: 60
Protein: 2 g
Carbs: 5 g
Fat: 4 g
Sat: 1 g

An unusual but tasty way to serve strawberries and it's a snap to make. Try adding blueberries and grapes for another variation.

2 tablespoons orange juice, fresh squeezed
1 tablespoon white wine vinegar
2 teaspoons extra-virgin olive oil
2 bags (6 cups) salad greens
1 cup quartered strawberries
1/4 cup (1 ounce) crumbled French feta cheese

Combine first three ingredients in a small bowl and whisk together.

Place greens, strawberries and cheese in a large bowl and add orange juice mixture, tossing to coat.

grilled chicken and mandarin orange salad

This salad is a frequent meal at my household and is so easy to make. Just serve with a glass of sparkling mineral water and voilá!

2 cans mandarin oranges
sea salt, pepper
1 cup fresh orange juice
1/2 cup rice wine vinegar
4 boneless, skinless chicken breasts (3 ounces each)
6 cups baby spinach leaves
1/2 small red onion, thinly sliced

Serves 4
per portion
Calories: 273
Protein: 33 g
Carbs: 31 g
Fat: 4 g
Sat: 1 g

In a bowl, combine the liquid from the mandarin oranges with the fresh orange juice and vinegar. Season with salt and pepper.

Split the dressing into two bowls.

Marinate the chicken breasts in one bowl of the dressing for 15 minutes. Grill the chicken until done, about 5 minutes per side.

Toss the spinach leaves with the remaining bowl of dressing and arrange on chilled individual serving plates. Cut each chicken breast crosswise into slices and arrange them along with the oranges on top of the spinach. Strew each salad with the red onions and serve immediately.

tuna and white bean salad

Serves 4
per portion
Calories: 275
Protein: 31 g
Carbs: 24 g
Fat: 7 g
Sat: 1 g

This recipe can be found in almost any Italian trattoria. It's an example of fine, clean flavors—a specialty of Mediterranean cuisine.

Dressing:
3 tablespoons fresh lemon juice
1/2 teaspoon sea salt
1/4 teaspoon white pepper
1 teaspoon extra-virgin olive oil

Salad:
1 pound radicchio, leaves separated
One bag romaine lettuce or 2 large heads, torn
1 red bell pepper, quartered, stemmed and seeded
1 can tuna in oil (drain the oil and reserve for
    the dressing)
1 can (15 ounces) white cannellini beans, rinsed well
2 tablespoons fresh snipped chives
2 tablespoons fresh snipped dill
2 tablespoons Italian parsley, finely chopped
2 large shallots, coarsely chopped

In a small bowl, mix the lemon juice with the salt and pepper until dissolved. Drain the can of tuna and add the oil to the olive oil. Pour the oil in a steady stream while continuously whisking the lemon juice until emulsified.

Cut the radicchio leaves into strips and toss with the torn romaine leaves. Dice the bell pepper, then add all the remaining ingredients.

Toss the salad, then add the dressing to coat.

soups

chayote soup with lemongrass and ginger

From a land of many islands comes a cuisine that mixes sweet and spicy tastes. Indonesians use tamarind, a sour tasting fruit from an evergreen tree that originated in Western Africa, instead of chayote. It is available in paste form in Asian and Latin markets. If you can't find fresh lemongrass, you can substitute 1/2 teaspoon lemon peel for each teaspoon of minced lemongrass. Kaffir lime leaves are fragrant and often sold frozen in Asian markets. You can substitute 1 tablespoon lime juice and 1/2 teaspoon grated lime peel for each lime leaf.

Serves 6
per portion
Calories: 38
Protein: 3 g
Carbs: 6 g
Fat: <1 g
Sat: 0 g

7 cups canned fat free, reduced sodium chicken broth
1 stalk fresh lemongrass, thinly sliced
   (about 2 teaspoons)
1 1-inch piece fresh ginger, sliced
3 fresh kaffir lime leaves
1/2 cinnamon Ceylon cinnamon stick (see Resources)
1/2 teaspoon ground nutmeg
1/4 teaspoon cayenne pepper
2 chayotes, peeled, rinsed, quartered, cored,
   thinly sliced crosswise
1/4 cup fresh lime juice
3/4 cup chopped fresh Italian parsley

Combine first 7 ingredients in a large pot and bring to a boil. Reduce heat and simmer 10 minutes to blend flavors. Strain liquid into bowl; return to same pot. Discard solids in strainer.

Bring liquid in pot to boil. Add chayotes; reduce heat and simmer until it is crisp-tender, about 7 minutes. Stir in lemon juice and parsley. Serve hot or chilled.

chilled cherry soup

Serves 4
per portion
Calories: 122
Protein: 4 g
Carbs: 22 g
Fat: 3 g
Sat: 1 g

This is a great way to use soy in your diet with this refreshing, colorful soup. Save a few cherries to serve on top.

1 cup apple juice
1 cup pitted, fresh cherries
1 cup unsweetened soy milk
1 stick cinnamon, preferably Ceylon or Mexican

Combine all the ingredients except the cinnamon stick in the blender. Pour the mixture into a saucepan and bring to a simmer over low heat. Add the cinnamon stick and cook an additional 2 to 3 minutes, until thick. Remove the cinnamon stick and chill until cold.

chilled cantaloupe and mint soup

Serves 4
per portion
Calories: 104
Protein: 4 g
Carbs: 15 g
Fat: 1 g
Sat: 0 g

This soup is wonderful in the summertime when melons are in abundance. Try using spearmint instead of peppermint for a unique flavor. If you want to get fancy, make another version with honeydew melons and pour the two into the same dish side by side for a real treat.

1 medium cantaloupe
1 1/2 tablespoons fresh mint
1 cup yogurt, low fat
1/2 cup dry white wine

Puree the cantaloupe and mint in a blender.
Pour into a bowl and mix with the yogurt and wine.
Chill overnight.

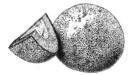

chilled chick pea, tomato and yogurt soup

Matthew Kenney of Mezze in New York serves this wonderful soup in the summer when the tomatoes are ripe and the afternoons long on sunshine. Chick peas are an ideal thickener for soup and they lose little of their nutty flavor when canned.

6 large, ripe tomatoes, peeled and seeded
2 teaspoons extra-virgin olive oil
2 cloves garlic, minced
1 teaspoon ground cardamom
1 teaspoon ground cumin
1 teaspoon ground ginger
2 cups canned chick peas, rinsed and drained
1 cup low-fat yogurt
sea salt, pepper
12 cilantro leaves, thinly sliced

Serves 4
per portion
Calories: 225
Protein: 10 g
Carbs: 37 g
Fat: 5 g
Sat: 1 g

Chop the tomatoes and set aside. Put the olive oil in a 4 quart saucepan over medium heat. Add the garlic and cook for 2 minutes, stirring to avoid burning. Add the tomatoes, cardamom, cumin and ginger and cook, uncovered for 15 minutes, or until the released tomato juices start to thicken.

Transfer the tomato-spice mixture to a food processor or blender and puree. Add the chick peas, 1/2 cup at a time, pulsing after each addition. The mixture should have a coarse texture. Pour into a bowl, stir in the yogurt and season with salt and pepper to taste. Refrigerate for at least 1 1/2 hours to overnight.

To serve, divide the soup among 4 chilled bowls and sprinkle with the cilantro.

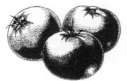

cream of bell pepper soup

Serves 4
per portion
Calories: 94
Protein: 3 g
Carbs: 7 g
Fat: 6 g
Sat: 2 g

With peppers coming in so many colors, you can make a rainbow of colored soups with this easy, quick recipe.

2 1/2 pounds single colored bell peppers
    (red, green, yellow, orange, purple)
2 teaspoons extra-virgin olive oil
1 cup chopped shallots
2 garlic cloves, minced
1 tablespoon chopped fresh thyme
3 cups or more canned vegetable broth
1/2 cup half and half
2 teaspoons red wine vinegar
1/2 teaspoon cayenne pepper
fresh basil, sliced or chiffonade

Char peppers over a gas flame or in a broiler until blackened on all sides. Enclose in a paper bag and let stand 10 minutes. Peel, seed and slice peppers.

Heat oil in a heavy large saucepan over medium heat. Add shallots, garlic and thyme and saute for 3 minutes. Add 3 cups of broth and all but 4 slices of roasted pepper. Simmer uncovered until peppers are very soft, about 20 minutes. Let cool 15 minutes.

Working in batches, puree the soup in a food processor until smooth. Return to the same pot and add half and half, vinegar and cayenne pepper. Rewarm the soup, thinning with additional broth as necessary and season with salt and pepper to taste. Garnish with a pepper strip and basil.

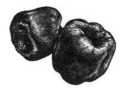

fennel and lemon soup

I am always looking for ways to serve unusual vegetables, and this one for fennel is easy, fast and delicious. It can be served either hot or chilled. Save some of the fennel leaves for garnish.

1 teaspoon extra-virgin olive oil
1 white onion, chopped
2 fennel bulbs, thinly sliced
2 1/2 cups chicken stock
1 cup milk 2%
sea salt, pepper
1 lemon, zested and juiced

Serves 4
per portion
Calories: 75
Protein: 4 g
Carbs: 10 g
Fat: 2 g
Sat: 1 g

Heat the skillet dry on high heat, then add the olive oil. Immediately reduce heat and add the onions. Cook over low heat for 5 minutes or until soft. Stir in the fennel pieces.

Add the stock and lemon zest and bring to a boil. Reduce the heat, cover and simmer for 20 minutes or until fennel is tender.

Transfer to a food processor and process until smooth. Add enough milk to give the desired consistency and season with salt and pepper. Stir in the lemon juice just before serving and garnish with some fennel leaves.

tomato and pumpkin soup

My grandmother was a Canadian wheat farmer's wife and she often served soup for breakfast. This unique take on a winter soup will have you in a "field of dreams" before you know it.

2 cups white onions, chopped
1 teaspoon canola oil
1/2 teaspoon nutmeg
1 can (14 1/2 oz.) pumpkin (not the one for pie)
1 can (14 1/2 oz.) Muir Glen organic tomatoes, chopped
1/4 cup finely chopped parsley
4 cups fat free, reduced sodium chicken stock
1 cup non-fat yogurt
6 oz tofu
sea salt, pepper to taste

Serves 8
per portion
Calories: 110
Protein: 8 g
Carbs: 14 g
Fat: 3 g
Sat: 0 g

Heat the skillet dry on high heat, then add the oil and saute the onions on medium heat until limp and translucent.

Add nutmeg, pumpkin, tomatoes, parsley and chicken stock and simmer for 5 minutes.

Add the yogurt and tofu, puree and season to taste.

name your own vegetable soup

Serves 8
per portion
Calories: 87
Protein: 8 g
Carbs: 10 g
Fat: 3 g
Sat: 0 g

Asparagus is plentiful on the California coast and when it's in season I make use of every part. This soup can be turned into whatever you wish merely by using two pounds of fresh something.

2 cups fat free, reduced sodium chicken stock
3 cups water
1 pound yellow onions, chopped
3 cloves garlic, coarsely chopped
1 teaspoon extra-virgin olive oil
2 pounds fresh *something*
   (either asparagus, spinach, broccoli)
6 oz tofu
sea salt, white pepper
2 tablespoons fresh tarragon, minced

Place the stock and water into a large pot and bring to a boil.

Heat a skillet dry on high heat, then add the oil and saute the onions and garlic over medium heat until soft. Add the broccoli and season with the salt and pepper. Continue to saute the broccoli until it is bright green and starting to soften. Do not burn the onions and garlic.

Empty the vegetable mixture into the boiling stockpot and cover. Return to a boil then uncover and boil for 5 to 10 minutes, being sure not to make the broccoli lose its color.

Remove from the heat, add the tofu and puree. Add the tarragon and serve after correcting the seasoning.

thai shrimp broth with lemongrass, chili and ginger

I often frequent the numerous Thai restaurants in my area and enjoy a bowlful of this heavenly soup whenever I can. Just don a cooley hat and imagine yourself floating on a sampan in Bangkok Harbor.

Serves 4
per portion
Calories: 121
Protein: 20 g
Carbs: 2 g
Fat: 3 g
Sat: 1 g

1/2 pound uncooked, large shrimp
4 14-1/2-ounce cans fat free, reduced sodium
    chicken broth
8 thin slices fresh lemongrass
2 tablespoons finely chopped ginger
1 tablespoon minced garlic
1 tablespoon finely chopped fresh basil
1 tablespoon finely chopped fresh mint
1 tablespoon finely chopped cilantro
1 small serrano chili, stemmed,
    thinly sliced into rounds
1 teaspoon fresh lime juice
4 thin lime slices

Peel and devein shrimp; reserve shells. Halve shrimp lengthwise and transfer to a small bowl. Cover and chill.

Combine reserved shrimp shells, broth and next 3 ingredients in a large pot. Bring to a boil. Reduce heat; simmer uncovered 20 minutes to blend flavors, stirring and skimming surface occasionally.

Strain broth into a large bowl, pressing on the solids with the back of a spoon to release as much liquid as possible; discard solids. Return broth to the pot. Bring to a simmer. Remove the heat and add the shrimp, herbs, chili and lime juice. Cover and let stand until shrimp are opaque, stirring once, about 2 minutes.

Ladle into bowls. Garnish with lime wedges.

seafood

orange roughy with orange, caper and olive sauce

Serves 4
per portion
Calories: 190
Protein: 14 g
Carbs: 13 g
Fat: 9 g
Sat: <1 g

This fish has a wonderful texture when baked with this sauce. By using a very hot oven, the fish remains moist and flaky.

1 orange
1/2 cup finely chopped seeded plum tomatoes
1/4 cup fresh orange juice
3 tablespoons minced red onion
1-1/2 tablespoons fresh lemon juice
2 teaspoons extra-virgin olive oil
5 minced Kalamata olives
1 tablespoon chopped, drained capers
1 teaspoon chopped fresh rosemary
4 3-ounce orange roughy fillets

Preheat oven to 500 degrees. Remove peel and white pith from orange. Cut twenty 2-inch-long, 1/8-inch wide strips of orange peel and reserve. Chop orange; place in a small, non-metallic bowl. Add tomatoes, onion, lemon juice, olive oil, olives, capers and rosemary to the chopped orange; stir to blend. Season with salt and pepper to taste.

Spray a glass baking dish with olive oil and arrange the fish in it. Sprinkle orange strips evenly over fish. Season with salt and pepper.

Bake until fish is opaque in center, about 10 minutes.

Spoon sauce over fish and serve.

ginger shrimp in napa cabbage

This recipe demonstrates how useful cabbage leaves can be as a wrap for shrimp, beef or chicken dishes. Like grape leaves, they are low in calories yet high in fiber.

One unpeeled 4-inch piece of fresh ginger
1 teaspoon sea salt
4 cups water
24 medium shrimp, peeled and deveined
12 Napa cabbage leaves, halved lengthwise,
    ribs removed
2 teaspoons Asian black bean sauce
1/2 cup radish sprouts

Makes 12 wraps
per wrap
Calories: 54
Protein: 12 g
Carbs: 1 g
Fat: 1 g
Sat: <1 g

In a food processor, finely chop the ginger. Transfer to a saucepan, add the salt and water and bring to a boil. Simmer over moderate heat for 10 minutes. Strain the ginger broth through a fine sieve, discarding the ginger. Return the broth to the pan and bring to a boil. Add the shrimp and cook over high heat until just opaque, about 1 minute. Remove the shrimp to a plate with a slotted spoon and let cool. Let the cooking liquid cool too, then add the shrimp and refirgerate until chilled, at least 30 minutes. Drain the shrimp and pat dry.

In a large pot of boiling water, cook the cabbage until tender, about 2 minutes. Drain and let cool under running water, then dry the cabbage leaves thoroughly with paper towels.

Cut the cabbage into 6-by-1-inch strips. Set a shrimp at one end of a cabbage strip, top with a scant teaspoon of the black bean sauce and a few of the sprouts and roll up the shrimp in the cabbage strip. Repeat with the remaining ingredients.

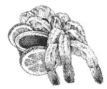

halibut with artichokes, zucchini and tomatoes

Serves 2
per portion
Calories: 208
Protein: 27 g
Carbs: 18 g
Fat: 3 g
Sat: <1 g

This dish is quick and simple. Try using sea bass or orange roughy if halibut is not fresh.

1 6-ounce jar marinated artichoke hearts
2 3-ounce halibut fillets
8 ounces plum tomatoes, chopped
1 zucchini, cut into rounds
3 tablespoons chopped, fresh basil
2 garlic cloves, minced
3/4 bottle clam juice

Preheat oven to 475 degrees. Drain marinade from artichokes into a 9-inch diameter glass pie dish. Add fish; turn to coat with marinade. Sprinkle fish with salt and pepper. Scatter artichokes, tomatoes, zucchini, basil and garlic around fish. Pour clam juice over the fish and bake until fish is just opaque in the center, about 20 minutes.

seared black scallops

Serves 2
per portion
Calories: 208
Protein: 27 g
Carbs: 18 g
Fat: 3 g
Sat: <1 g

I use the black seeds, called Nigella, common to Morocco and India. It gives a wonderful color contrast to the white scallops and imparts a sweet taste.

3 tablespoons Nigella or black seeds (see Resources)
1 1/2 teaspoon sea salt
1/8 teaspoon freshly ground black pepper
6 large sea scallops (about 5 ounces)
2 teaspoons extra-virgin olive oil

In a small bowl stir together the seeds, salt and pepper. Trim the scallops of any tough muscle that is attached on the side and pat scallops dry. Dip flat sides of each scallop in the seed mixture.

In a 12-inch nonstick skillet heat oil over moderately high heat until hot but not smoking and saute scallops on the flat sides until the seeds are fragrant and scallops are just cooked through, about 4 minutes total.

mussels in chipotle chili broth

One year, for my birthday, friends took me to three restaurants in one night, where we ate mussels prepared in different styles. This recipe, from Rocking Horse Café Mexicano, is a great way to serve the new, farm raised mussels. Do like the natives and use the shell to scoop up the spicy broth before sucking the mussels right off. ¡Ay Caramba!

Serves 4
per portion
Calories: 178
Protein: 15 g
Carbs: 11 g
Fat: 5 g
Sat: 1 g

2 teaspoons peanut oil
3 garlic cloves, minced
1 tablespoon minced canned chipotle chilis
3 pounds mussels, (12 ounces meat only)
    scrubbed and debearded*
1/2 cup dry white wine
1 cup fish stock or bottled clam juice
6 plum tomatoes, coarsely chopped
5 Kalamata olives, pitted and sliced
4 tablespoons chopped fresh cilantro
sea salt to taste

Heat a large, heavy pot over medium-high heat and add oil. Add garlic and saute for 30 seconds (do not burn the garlic). Mix in the chipotle chilis, then add the wine, mussels and stock; cover and cook 4 minutes. Mix in tomatoes, olives and 2 tbsp. cilantro. Cover and cook until mussels open, about 3 minutes longer. Discard any mussels that don't open, then season to taste with sea salt.

Transfer mussels and broth to individual bowls and sprinkle with the remaining 2 tbsp. of cilantro.

* To check if your mussels are alive, put them in the freezer for 5 minutes. Any mussels that remain open should be discarded.

sea bass with chili and saffron

Sea bass is a popular white fish with excellent texture. It takes on new flavors when treated with this Near East recipe.

Serves 4
per portion
Calories: 261
Protein: 27 g
Carbs: 22 g
Fat: 7 g   Sat: 1 g

2 red bell peppers
8 Italian tomatoes, peeled*
5 tablespoons chopped cilantro

2 cloves garlic, chopped
1/2 teaspoon ground cumin
1/2 teaspoon ancho chili powder
1/4 teaspoon saffron threads
1 teaspoon paprika
sea salt, pepper
pinch of cayenne
2 teaspoons spicy olive oil
4 filets of sea bass, 4 ounces each
1/2 cup clam juice or fish stock
1 cup chick peas, rinsed and drained
harissa (optional—see Resources)

Char the peppers on the stove over a hot flame. If you have an electric cooktop, then preheat the broiler and put the peppers on a sheet pan lined with foil and broil for about 15 minutes, turning once or twice to ensure they blister and blacken. Place in a paper bag and let cool. Peel, seed and cut into 1/2 inch wide strips. Set aside. Cut the tomatoes lengthwise and into eighths. Set aside.

Preheat the oven to 350 degrees.

In a small bowl, combine 2 tablespoons of the cilantro, garlic, cumin, chilis, saffron, paprika, salt, black pepper, cayenne and olive oil. If you wish a truly spicy version, add a dab of harissa. Rub each fillet with the mixture and add the remainder to the stock. Warm the stock in a small saucepan.

Place the fish tightly in a baking dish. Spread the chick peas, tomatoes, and peppers evenly on top of the fish. Pour the stock over and cover with foil. Bake for 15 minutes, remove the foil and bake 5 more minutes. Transfer the fish to a platter, surround with the vegetables and pour the cooking liquid over the fish. Sprinkle with the remaining cilantro.

To peel tomatoes, drop them in boiling water for 30 seconds, then drop in ice water. The peel will slip right off.

provencal style lemon sole

This dish is quick to make and works equally well with halibut or even scallops if you are unable to find fresh lemon sole.

2 navel oranges
2 teaspoons extra-virgin olive oil
1 large red onion, thinly sliced
1 tablespoon thinly sliced garlic
3/4 cup (6 ounces) canned tomatoes, chopped
3/4 cup dry white wine
5 Kalamata olives, pitted and cut into thin slivers
4 4-ounce lemon sole fillets
Chives, cut into 1 1/2-inch lengths for garnish

Using a sharp knife, peel the oranges, removing all of the white pith and cut between the membranes to release the orange sections into a medium bowl.

Heat the oil in a large, deep skillet. Add the onion and garlic and cook over moderate heat until lightly browned, about 5 minutes. Stir in the tomatoes and wine and season with salt and pepper. Cook until the liquid is slightly reduced, about 4 minutes. Add the olives and set the fish fillets on top in a single layer. Season with salt and pepper, cover and cook until the fillets easily flake, about 7 minutes. Carefully transfer the fish to a platter.

Stir the oranges into the sauce and spoon the sauce onto plates. Set the fillets on top. Garnish with the chives and serve at once.

Serves 4
per portion
Calories: 210
Protein: 23 g
Carbs: 13 g
Fat: 4 g
Sat: 1 g

shrimp with two mushrooms

While visiting the island of Santorini, I tasted this wonderful dish made with two mushrooms and freshly caught shrimp. The smell of the salt air still lingers in my mind whenever I make this.

Serves 4
per portion
Calories: 165
Protein: 24 g
Carbs: 7 g
Fat: 5 g   Sat: 1 g

1/2 cup dried porcini mushrooms (about 1/2 ounce)
1/2 cup dried morel mushrooms (about 1/2 ounce)
2 cups hot water
2 teaspoons extra-virgin olive oil
1 pound large, uncooked, cleaned shrimp
1/3 cup Madeira
2 tablespoons chopped fresh Italian parsley
2 teaspoons sesame seeds

Place dried mushrooms in a bowl and cover with the hot water. Let stand for 30 minutes, or until soft. Using a slotted spoon, transfer the mushrooms to a small bowl, reserving the soaking liquid.

Heat a large, nonstick pan over moderate heat and add the olive oil. Add mushrooms and saute 2 minutes. Add shrimp; saute 1 minute. Add the wine and simmer until almost all the liquid evaporates, about 1 minute. Add 1/3 cup reserved mushroom soaking liquid (leave the sediment behind). Saute until shrimp are just cooked through, about 2 minutes.

Mix in the parsley and divide among 4 plates. Sprinkle with the sesame seeds.

sear-roasted halibut

Serves 2
per portion
Calories: 183
Protein: 35 g
Carbs: 0 g
Fat: 4 g
Sat: <1 g

12 ounces fresh halibut fillet, about 1 inch thick
sea salt or seasoning of your choice

Heat the oven to 500 degrees for 20 minutes. Heat the roasting pan dry on high heat until you can't hold your hand over the pan for longer than the count of 3. Season the halibut with sea salt on both sides or with a seasoning mixture of your choice. Spray the roasting pan with olive oil and place the halibut on the pan to sear one side. This will take about 1 minute. Turn the halibut over and immediately place the pan in the oven and roast for 8 minutes.

tu tu tun lodge grilled salmon

As a neighbor of Dirk and Laurie van Zantes, owners of the Tu Tu Tun Lodge, I look forward to the day whole, fresh caught Rogue River salmon are served. Laurie uses fresh applewood from their orchard, but wood chips work nicely as well. It's worth buying a whole salmon, so invite lots of friends to share in this wonderful feast.

Serves 12
per portion
Calories: 250
Protein: 32 g
Carbs: <1 g
Fat: 12 g
Sat: 2 g

1 teaspoon extra-virgin olive oil
3 1/2 - 4 pound salmon fillet with the skin
1/4 cup dry white wine
2 teaspoons fresh lemon juice
2 teaspoons minced fresh garlic
1 tablespoon finely chopped fresh parsley
2 teaspoons fresh thyme leaves
sea salt, pepper to taste

Prepare a grill by opening vents and filling a chimney starter with charcoal and light. (Do not use lighter fluid). Charcoal will be ready when it is lightly coated with gray ash, 15 to 20 minutes. Mound lighted charcoal on opposite sides of grill bottom, leaving the middle clear. Spread apple branches that have been soaked in water overnight over the charcoal and position the rack. When wood begins to smoke, in about 2 minutes, grill is ready.

While the charcoal is lighting, use heavy duty foil in 2 layers and make a shallow baking pan just large enough to fit the salmon and put the pan on a large baking sheet to stabilize it. Spray foil with oil and put the salmon, skin side down, on foil. Pour wine and lemon juice evenly over the salmon and spray a small amount of oil over the fish. Sprinkle garlic, parsley, thyme, salt and pepper over the fish and carefully slide the foil package onto the center of the grill and cover. Grill salmon over indirect heat, without turning, until just cooked through, about 25 to 30 minutes.

baked basque cod

Serves 4
per portion
Calories: 140
Protein: 21 g
Carbs: 6 g
Fat: 3 g
Sat: 1 g

Cod is a simple fish widely available in the Basque region of Spain and is a mainstay in their cooking. Try making a mixture of vegetables available in the fresh produce section for a different variation. This also works well with red snapper.

2 teaspoons extra-virgin olive oil
1 green pepper, diced
1 white onion, finely chopped
2 tomatoes, peeled and diced
1 garlic clove, crushed
2 teaspoons fresh basil
4 cod fillets, skinned, approximately 4 ounces each
Juice of 1/2 lemon
sea salt, pepper
lemon slices for garnish

Heat oven to 375 degrees. Brush four large squares of foil with a little oil.

Mix together the bell pepper, onion, tomatoes, garlic and basil. Put a fillet in the center of each foil piece and top with the mixture.

Drizzle with lemon juice and the remaining oil and season with salt and pepper. Fold the foil into parcels and place on a baking sheet in the oven for 20 minutes or until the fish flakes easily.

Unwrap the foil and transfer the fish, vegetables and cooking juices onto serving plates.

Garnish with lemon slices and serve.

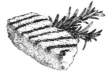

poultry

calcutta chicken in spinach and yogurt sauce

This dish is made with seasoning characteristic of the west Bengal region of India. For a truly authentic taste, use mustard oil instead of canola. Make sure you heat the mustard oil to the smoking point and let it smoke for 3 to 5 seconds before adding the ingredients. This tempers its pungency.

12 ounces boneless, skinless chicken breasts
1 bunch baby spinach leaves
1 medium white onion
4 large garlic cloves
1 small serrano chile
1 1-inch piece fresh gingerroot
1/2 teaspoon brown or black mustard seeds
1 tablespoon mustard oil or canola oil
2 teaspoons ground coriander seeds
1 cup plain, whole milk yogurt
1 teaspoon sea salt

Serves 4
per portion
Calories: 235
Protein: 29 g
Carbs: 10 g
Fat: 8 g
Sat: 2 g

Chop the chicken breasts into pieces. Discard the stems from the baby spinach leaves and chop enough spinach to measure 2 cups. Chop the onion and mince the garlic and the chile pepper. Peel the gingerroot and mince. With a spice grinder, coarsely grind the mustard seeds.

In a heavy 12-inch skillet, heat the mustard oil over high heat until smoking, then reduce the heat to moderate and cook the onion, garlic, serrano, gingerroot and mustard seeds, stirring until the onion begins to brown. Add the coriander and cook, stirring, 1 minute. Stir in the spinach and cook until it begins to wilt, about 30 seconds. Gradually add yogurt, stirring until well combined. Stir in the chicken pieces, salt and simmer the mixture until the chicken is cooked, about 5 minutes.

chicken, tofu and watercress stir-fry

Serves 6
per portion
Calories: 159
Protein: 26 g
Carbs: 1 g
Fat: 5 g
Sat: 1 g

Another fast, easy way to incorporate soy into your diet. Remember to let the wok heat up until you can't hold your hand over the pan longer than 3 seconds. Just add the oil and you'll be wokking the fat out of your diet.

1 teaspoon peanut oil
12 ounces boneless, skinless chicken breast,
    cut into strips
3 ounces firm tofu, cut into 1/2-inch cubes
4 tablespoons Chinese oyster sauce
1 cup water or fat free, reduced sodium chicken broth
4 cups watercress, cut into 2-inch lengths

Heat the pan over high heat dry, then add peanut oil and immediately add the chicken pieces and tofu cubes, stirring often to brown all sides. Combine the oyster sauce with the water or broth and stir the liquid into the stir-fry. Once it is hot, add the watercress and reduce the heat to low. Cover the pan and cook for one minute or until the chicken is cooked through and the watercress has wilted.

roasted turkey breast

per portion
3 ounces
Calories: 47
Protein: 10 g
Carbs: 0 g
Fat: <1 g
Sat: 0 g

This is so simple and delicious, you'll be wishing it was Thanksgiving every day.

1 turkey breast
California BBQ seasoning (p. 121)

Heat the oven to 350 degrees.
Take the turkey breast and season under the skin with the California BBQ seasoning. Place it in an oven-proof pan and roast for one hour.

chicken with spiced yogurt marinade

This dish is popular in Afghanistan where it works equally well with lamb and chicken. The perfume of saffron contrasts nicely with the piquancy of lemon juice and garlic in this tangy marinade. Don't use boneless chicken as it will not remain juicy on the grill.

2 cups whole milk yogurt
2 tablespoons fresh lemon juice
4 garlic cloves, minced
1 medium yellow onion, minced
2 teaspoons ground coriander
1 teaspoon ground cumin
2 teaspoons sea salt
1 teaspoon white pepper
1/2 teaspoon saffron threads, crumbled
1/2 teaspoon cinnamon
8 chicken breasts and thighs, bone in, including skin

Serves 8
per portion
Calories: 211
Protein: 21 g
Carbs: 4 g
Fat: 11 g
Sat: 3 g

In a bowl combine the yogurt, lemon juice, garlic, onion, coriander, cumin, salt, pepper, saffron and cinnamon. Stir well to blend.

Place the chicken pieces in a large glass or ceramic dish and pour the marinade on top. Let marinate 4 hours or overnight.

Light a grill and cook the chicken pieces over a medium-hot fire, turning often, until lightly charred on both sides and just cooked through, about 10 minutes per side.

lemon tarragon chicken

A simple, classic French dish that takes so little time, but makes a great impression.

2 medium-size lemons
1 tablespoon chopped fresh tarragon or 1/2 teaspoon dried
2 teaspoons olive oil
sea salt, pepper
1 garlic clove, minced
4 small skinless, boneless chicken breasts, 3 ounces each

Serves 4
per portion
Calories: 149
Protein: 24 g
Carbs: 0 g
Fat: 5 g
Sat: 1 g

From 1 lemon, grate enough peel to equal 2 teaspoons. Thinly slice half of second lemon; reserve slices for garnish. Squeeze juice from remaining 3 lemon halves into small bowl. Stir in lemon peel, tarragon, olive oil, salt, pepper, and garlic.

Toss chicken breast halves with the lemon juice mixture. Heat skillet dry over high heat.

Place chicken breast halves in hot skillet; cook 5 minutes, brushing with remaining lemon-juice mixture in bowl. Turn chicken over and cook 5 minutes longer until juices run clear when thickest part of chicken breast is pierced with a knife. Garnish with lemon slices.

chicken breasts with thyme-lemon marinade

Serves 4
per portion
Calories: 132
Protein: 24 g
Carbs: 1 g
Fat: 3 g
Sat: 1 g

This dish is a regular at my house. It's quick, easy and very low in fat and calories. Serve it with steamed, fresh broccoli studded with toasted almonds for a real treat!

4 3-ounce boneless, skinless chicken breasts
3 tablespoons fresh lemon juice
1 tablespoon chopped fresh thyme or 1 teaspoon dried
2 teaspoons grated lemon peel
2 garlic cloves, pressed

Place chicken breasts in a plastic bag.

Mix the lemon juice, thyme, lemon peel and garlic in small bowl.

Pour the mixture over the chicken and massage the bag to cover all the chicken. Refrigerate one hour or up to one day.

Remove the chicken from the bag and grill for 3 minutes per side.

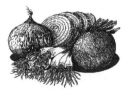

indian turkey cutlets

This is a great way to use those turkey slices in the meat department. Be careful not to soak them in the yogurt or they will take on a mealy characteristic.

Serves 6
per portion
Calories: 153
Protein: 28 g
Carbs: 3 g
Fat: 3 g
Sat: 1 g

2 large limes
1/3 cup plain low-fat yogurt
2 teaspoons canola oil
2 teaspoons minced, peeled gingerroot
1 teaspoon ground cumin
1 teaspoon ground coriander
sea salt
1 garlic clove, crushed with garlic press
1 1/2 pounds turkey cutlets
cilantro sprigs for garnish

From 1 lime, grate 1 teaspoon peel and squeeze 1 tablespoon juice. Cut the remaining lime into wedges; reserve wedges for squeezing juice over cooked cutlets. In large bowl, mix lime peel, lime juice, yogurt, canola oil, gingerroot, cumin, coriander, salt, and garlic until blended.

Just before grilling, add turkey cutlets to bowl with yogurt mixture, stirring to coat cutlets.

Place turkey cutlets on grill over medium heat. Cook cutlets 5 to 7 minutes until they just lose their pink color throughout. Serve with lime wedges. Garnish with cilantro sprigs.

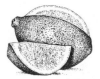

meat

moorish spicy lamb kebabs

Serves 8
per portion
Calories: 110
Protein: 12 g
Carbs: 1 g
Fat: 6 g
Sat: 2 g

This is a heavily seasoned meat mixture that is best cooked over a charcoal grill. I was served this dish in Istanbul, while watching the sun gently lower into the sea behind the Blue Mosque.

2 garlic cloves, sliced
sea salt and black pepper
1 teaspoon coriander seeds
3/4 teaspoon paprika
3/4 teaspoon cumin seeds
1/2 teaspoon dried thyme
1/4 teaspoon crushed red pepper flakes
1 teaspoon curry powder
6 teaspoons olive oil
2 tablespoons lemon juice
1 tablespoon chopped fresh parsley
1 pound lean lamb, pork or beef,
      cut into 3/4 inch cubes

In a mortar, pound the garlic with a pinch of salt to make a paste.

Heat a skillet dry on high, then toast coriander seeds, cumin seeds, thyme, crushed red pepper and curry powder until hot and aromatic, about 30 seconds. Remove from the pan and put the mixture into a spice grinder until reduced to a fine powder.

In a bowl, combine the garlic, spices, olive oil, lemon juice, parsley, 3/4 teaspoon salt, pepper and the meat cubes. Toss well to coat completely and let marinate several hours, mixing occasionally.

Skewer the meat and grill over the coals, turning every 2-3 minutes, until well browned and still juicy, about 10 to 15 minutes. Baste occasionally with the marinade. Serve immediately.

filet mignon with castello blue cheese

This is one of my favorite ways to top a great filet. Just put a dab of this Danish triple cream blue cheese on a hot, grilled filet and watch it melt away your day. I roast the filet after searing on a hot griddle to insure the meat remains moist as it cooks.

1 3-ounce filet mignon
1/2 ounce Blue Castello triple cream cheese

Heat your oven to 500 degrees.

Heat an oven-tolerant grill on high, then sear the filet on one side, turning with tongs to make a cross hatch pattern on one side of the meat.

Turn the meat over and immediately place in the 500 degree oven. Cook 3 minutes for medium rare.

Serve the meat on a dish topped with a dab of cheese. Wait for it to melt before eating.

Serves 1
per portion
Calories: 181
Protein: 19 g
Carbs: 0 g
Fat: 12 g
Sat: 6 g

spicy beef with basil

There are numerous basils to choose from, but this dish cries out for its native Vietnamese basil, called holy basil. You can substitute Italian basil but you need to add mint leaves to try and approximate the unique flavor of holy basil. Look for it in any Far Eastern market.

1 teaspoon white peppercorns
2 garlic cloves, finely chopped
1 1/2 tablespoons coarsely chopped cilantro
1 tablespoon minced fresh ginger
2 Thai or serrano chilis, minced
1 1/2 teaspoons finely grated lime zest
1 teaspoon sea salt
1 teaspoon canola oil
8 ounces lean top round steak, cut into strips
2 tablespoons reduce sodium soy sauce
1 cup holy basil leaves, or 1/2 cup Italian basil
    and 1/2 cup mint leaves

Serves 4
per portion
Calories: 108
Protein: 14 g
Carbs: 3 g
Fat: 4 g
Sat: 1 g

Heat a small skillet dry on high heat, then toast the peppercorns until fragrant, about 1 minute. Transfer to a spice grinder and coarsely crush. In a bowl, add the garlic, cilantro, ginger, chilis, lime zest, peppercorns, sea salt and pound to a coarse paste.

Heat the skillet on high, then add the oil and reduce the heat to medium. Add the beef and stir-fry until cooked through, about 2 minutes. Stir in the soy sauce and transfer to serving bowls. Top with the basil.

cuban grilled skirt steak

Serves 2
per portion
Calories: 159
Protein: 15 g
Carbs: 7 g
Fat: 8 g
Sat: 4 g

For this technique, it is easiest to partially freeze the skirt steak in order to slice it thin enough. If you substitute flank steak for skirt, you will need to slice it very thin or it will be tough.

1/2 small white onion, diced
1 serrano or jalapeno chili, diced
1/4 cup cilantro, chopped
1 garlic clove, minced
1 lime, juiced
2 teaspoons peanut oil
1/3 pound skirt steak

Combine onion, chili, cilantro, garlic and the juice of one lime in a non-reactive pan.

Partially freeze the skirt steak which has been trimmed of all fat. Using a very sharp knife, cut the steak in half horizontally. This may be done in sections, but the result will be a very thin cut of meat.

Combine the meat sections in the marinade for 15 minutes.

On a hot grill, quickly cook the meat until the edges are charred, turning only once. The meat will be medium rare inside.

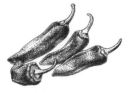

pork chops with chipotle marinade

Today's pork is leaner than ever and lowers cholesterol better than poultry. If you like a fiery, hot dish, this seasoning will do the trick.

2 tablespoons canned chipotle peppers,
    including sauce
2 garlic cloves, crushed
1 3-inch strip of orange zest
1/4 cup fresh orange juice
1 tablespoon fresh lime juice
1/2 tablespoon red wine vinegar
3/4 teaspoon tomato paste
1/4 teaspoon dried Mexican oregano
1/4 teaspoon ground cumin
fresh pepper, sea salt to taste
2 3-ounce pork chops

Serves 2
per portion
Calories: 130
Protein: 18 g
Carbs: 6 g
Fat: 3 g
Sat: 1 g

In a small saucepan, combine the chipotles and their sauce with the garlic, orange zest, orange juice, lime juice, red wine vinegar, tomato paste, oregano, cumin and pepper. Simmer over high heat until reduced by one-third, about 3 minutes. Puree everything in a food processor until smooth. Let cool before using.

Place pork chops in a plastic bag and cover with the marinade. Refrigerate for 2 hours.

Grill on high heat for 5 minutes per side.

flank steak in adobo seasoning

---

1 1-1/2 pound flank steak, trimmed of any fat
3 to 4 cloves garlic, cut into slivers
adobo seasoning (pg. 120)

Serves 6
per portion
Calories: 135
Protein: 14 g
Carbs: <1 g
Fat: 8 g
Sat: 3 g

Take flank steak and lightly score the surface on both sides in a criss-cross diamond pattern. Make slits in the meat and insert the slivers of garlic. Rub both sides of the meat with the adobo seasoning and place in a plastic bag in the refrigerator overnight.

Cook over a hot grill until the steak is rare inside and charred on the outside, about 7 to 9 minutes. Slice meat thinly across the grain.

vegetables

leeks nicoise

Serves 4
per portion
Calories: 109
Protein: 2 g
Carbs: 12 g
Fat: 7 g
Sat: 1 g

Here's another way to get onions into your diet. Leeks may contain dirt so be sure to split them at the bottom, make two deep cuts into the root and rinse well under water. Use a mandolin to finely slice the onions.

2 teaspoons extra-virgin olive oil
1 onion, thinly sliced
8 small leeks, cleaned
3 tomatoes, peeled and cut into eighths
1 garlic clove, crushed
1 tablespoon fresh basil, chopped
1 tablespoon fresh parsley, chopped
8 black olives, pitted and halved
sea salt, pepper
basil leaves to garnish

Heat a skillet dry on high then add the oil. Immediately reduce the heat and add the onions, cooking for 5 minutes or until soft. Add the leeks and cook, turning until just beginning to brown.

Add tomatoes. Stir in garlic, basil, parsley, olives, salt and pepper. Cover and cook over low heat 15 to 20 minutes or until leeks are tender, turning from time to time.

Remove leeks with a slotted spoon and transfer to a warm serving dish. Boil sauce for 2 minutes or until reduced and thickened. Pour over leeks and serve with basil leaves for garnish. May be presented hot or at room temperature.

aztec zucchini

This recipe comes from Emma Gonzalez, an Aztec raised in the mountains of Oaxaca. This is one of her most requested dishes. Do not substitute the type of mint or the oil as the flavor will not be the same.

2 teaspoons peanut oil
2 cans (14 1/2 ounces) Muir Glen tomatoes
1 clove garlic, chopped
1/4 white onion chopped
1 pound zucchini, sliced on the diagonal
1 tablespoon dried or 1/4 cup fresh spearmint,
    chopped
1/2 bunch cilantro, chopped

Heat an iron skillet dry on high heat, then add the peanut oil. Saute the tomatoes, garlic and onions until limp using a wooden spoon.

Add the zucchini, spearmint and cilantro and lower the heat. Cover and set on a low simmer for 15 minutes.

Serves 6
per portion
Calories: 95
Protein: 3 g
Carbs: 18 g
Fat: 2 g
Sat: <1 g

cauliflower leek puree

A great way to serve cauliflower is to puree it, adding another vegetable for flavor. Be sure to use only the white and pale green parts of the leeks and clean them carefully.

6 cups cauliflower, cut into pieces
1 cup chopped leeks
1 can fat free, reduced sodium chicken broth
sea salt, pepper

Place cauliflower, leeks and chicken broth in a microwave-safe bowl. Cover with plastic wrap and microwave on high for 14 minutes, or until vegetables are soft.

Transfer the vegetables to a food processor and blend until smooth. Add any cooking broth by tablespoons to achieve desired thickness and season with salt and pepper.

Serves 8
per portion
Calories: 33
Protein: 2 g
Carbs: 6 g
Fat: <1 g
Sat: 0 g

balsamic roasted squash and apples

Serves 4
per portion
Calories: 109
Protein: 2 g
Carbs: 26 g
Fat: 1 g
Sat: <1 g

This is another dish that comes alive with the unique pairing of balsamic and reduced apple cider glaze. I think you will find this dish is well worth the effort.

1/2 cup balsamic vinegar
1 cup fat free, reduced sodium chicken broth
few sprigs thyme
1 tablespoon apple cider glaze (see page 123)
2 (1- to 1-1/4 pound) acorn squash, halved
nonstick spray
2 green apples, peeled and cut into eighths
sea salt, pepper

Set the oven for 425 degrees.

Combine the vinegar, broth and thyme. Bring to a boil, then reduce the heat and simmer until the liquid is reduced to about 1/3 cup, about 15 minutes. Add the tablespoon of apple cider glaze and stir.

Remove the seeds from the squash and arrange the squash cut-side up in a single layer on a baking pan sprayed with nonstick cooking spray. Add the apples and brush with the balsamic glaze. Season with salt and pepper.

Roast until tender, about 35 minutes, brushing squash several times with the glaze.

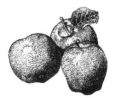

kabocha squash with tunisian flavors

Kabocha squash is a winter squash member that tastes sweet like pumpkin. It is used in Tunisia and Morocco. If you can't find it in your local grocery store, use butternut or pumpkin.

2 pounds kabocha squash
2 tablespoons water
1 head of garlic
1 teaspoon coriander
1/2 teaspoon cumin seeds
1/4 teaspoon caraway seeds
1 teaspoon sweet paprika
sea salt
pinch of cayenne
1 teaspoon fresh lemon juice

Serves 4
per portion
Calories: 50
Protein: 2 g
Carbs: 11 g
Fat: 1 g
Sat: 0 g

Preheat oven to 350 degrees. Cut the squash in half and scoop out the seeds. Set the halves, cut side down, on a lightly oiled baking sheet. Sprinkle the water on the pan. Pull the outer skin off the garlic, keeping the head intact. Wrap tightly in foil and place on the baking sheet. Bake until the squash is completely tender and the garlic feels soft, about 50 minutes. Let cool.

Scoop the squash flesh into the bowl of a food processor. Separate the garlic cloves and squeeze the pulp into the processor bowl.

In a small skillet, toast the coriander, cumin and caraway seeds over low heat until fragrant. Stir in the paprika. Transfer the spices to a mortar or spice grinder and let cool. Add 3/4 teaspoon salt and the cayenne and grind into a powder. Add half of the spice mix to the squash and process to a fine puree. Stir in more of the spice mix to taste. To serve, reheat the squash mixture in a pan sprayed with olive oil. Add the lemon juice and season with salt and pepper.

stir-fried bok choy

Serves 2
per portion
Calories: 29
Protein: 1 g
Carbs: 1 g
Fat: 2 g
Sat: <1 g

Known as Chinese cabbage, bok choy makes a wonderful vegetable to accompany pork dishes. Be sure and buy ones with dark green leaves as they contain lots of beta carotene. Here is an easy stir-fry version.

1 head bok choy
2 tablespoons water
1 1/2 teaspoons soy sauce, reduced salt
1 1/2 teaspoons oyster sauce
1 teaspoon peanut oil

Trim bok choy and cut crosswise into 1/4 inch slices.
In a bowl stir together water, soy and oyster sauces.
Heat dry a large heavy skillet or wok over high heat, then add oil and stir-fry boy choy for 2 minutes. Add the soy mixture and cook until crisp-tender, about 2 more minutes.

warm mixed greens

Serves 4
per portion
Calories: 87
Protein: 3 g
Carbs: 9 g
Fat: 6 g
Sat: 2 g

This is a delicious way to serve collard, kale, Swiss chard or mustard greens. For a slightly sweeter taste, add a tablespoon of reduced apple cider for a piquant flavor.

1 tablespoon unsalted butter
2 teaspoons extra-virgin olive oil
2 pounds braising greens trimmed and
    coarsely chopped
1 tablespoon reduced apple cider (p. 123)
2 tablespoons water
sea salt, pepper

In a large heavy saucepan, melt the butter in the olive oil. Add the greens, reduced apple cider and water and season with salt and pepper. Cover and cook over high heat until wilted and tender, about 2 to 3 minutes. Drain the greens and keep warm.

zucchini noodles with spicy tomato sauce

This is a fun dish. I used a Japanese mandolin that makes oodles of noodles out of any vegetable. For even more variety, alternate yellow and green squash. The splash of tomato sauce makes this dish "eye candy" for anyone lucky enough to have it placed before them.

Makes 2 1/2 cups
per 1/2 cup
Calories: 43
Protein: 1 g
Carbs: 6 g
Fat: 2 g
Sat: <1 g

Spicy Tomato Sauce
This will coat 1 pound of vegetable pasta
1 tablespoon extra-virgin olive oil
1/2 cup thinly sliced sweet onions
    (Vidalia, Walla Walla, Maui)
2 large garlic cloves, thinly sliced
2 14-1/2-ounce cans of Muir Glen peeled tomatoes
1/2 teaspoon crushed red pepper
sea salt
1 tablespoon minced spearmint

Heat a large skillet dry on high heat then add oil. Immediately lower the heat and add the onion and cook, stirring, until softened and just brown, about 5 minutes. Stir in the garlic and cook for 1 minute. Add the tomatoes with their juice and the crushed red pepper. Season with salt and cook, stirring, until thickened, about 20 minutes. Stir in the mint.

zucchini noodles

If you want to save time or don't have a Japanese mandolin, use spaghetti squash and bake according to directions. To save even more time and calories, blanch the "noodles" in boiling water for 2 minutes and drain.

Serves 4
per portion
Calories: 50
Protein: 1 g
Carbs: 4 g
Fat: 4 g
Sat: <1 g

1 tablespoon extra-virgin olive oil
1 1/2 teaspoons thyme leaves
1 teaspoon minced garlic
1 1/2 pounds zucchini, yellow squash,
    finely shredded into noodles
sea salt, pepper

In a large skillet, warm the olive oil and add half the thyme and all the garlic and cook over moderate heat for 1 minute. Add the zucchini and cook, stirring occasionally, until it just begins to lose its crunch, about 3 minutes. Season with salt and pepper.

Top with the spicy tomato sauce.

roasted sweet red peppers

Serves 4-6
per portion
Calories: 40
Protein: 1 g
Carbs: 4 g
Fat: 2 g
Sat: 0 g

I often make jars of roasted peppers to have on hand when I want a really great snack. They go especially well with goat cheese and basil.

4 to 6 medium red peppers
2 garlic cloves, minced
2 tablespoons red wine vinegar
2 teaspoons extra-virgin olive oil
sea salt
2 tablespoons chopped fresh basil

Roast the peppers over a flame until charred and blistered. Set in a paper bag and let cool. Remove the skins. Split the peppers in half and remove the seeds and inner membranes. Cut the peppers into wide strips.

Place in a bowl and toss with the garlic, vinegar, olive oil and salt to taste. Cover and refrigerate until ready to serve. Do not add the basil until ready to serve.

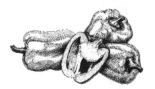

joel's asparagus bake

Joel is a very busy executive who finds time to cook only on the weekends. This is his easy, no holds barred approach for creating scrumptious, juicy asparagus every time. I like dipping it in soyamaise for vegetables (p. 132).

Extra-virgin olive oil in a pump
1 pound asparagus, cleaned and trimmed
sea salt

Heat the oven to 400 degrees. Prepare the asparagus and place them flat in a lightly oiled glass dish. Do not bunch them up. Sprinkle with sea salt, spray with some additional oil and cover with foil.

Place in the oven on the middle rack and roast for 10 minutes. Remove the foil and roast an additional 10 minutes.

Serves 2
per portion
Calories: 32
Protein: 6 g
Carbs: 3 g
Fat: <1 g
Sat: 0 g

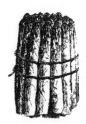

cereals, grains and beans

garbanzos with garlic and kale

Serves 6
per portion
Calories: 122
Protein: 6 g
Carbs: 22 g
Fat: 2 g
Sat: <1 g

During a trip to Hong Kong, I tasted this dish at a little sidewalk shop that was filled with locals. I think you will agree it has a unique, filling taste.

2 bunches kale or collard greens
1 teaspoon extra-virgin olive oil
4 cloves garlic
1 tablespoon minced gingerrroot
1 red chili pepper, finely chopped
2 tomatoes, coarsely chopped
1 15-ounce can garbanzo beans, including liquid
1 teaspoon reduced sodium soy sauce
1 teaspoon hoisin sauce

Wash the kale, remove the stems and chop the leaves.

Heat the oil in a large skillet and saute the garlic, gingerroot and pepper for 2 minutes.

Stir in the tomatoes and garbanzo beans with their liquid. Bring to a simmer and cook for 5 minutes.

Add the soy sauce, hoisin sauce and stir to mix. Spread the kale evenly over the top, then cover the pan and cook over medium heat, stirring occasionally, until the kale is tender, about 5 to 7 minutes. Do not overcook.

connemara irish oatmeal

My daughter and I took a trip to Ireland where we explored the countryside and frightened quite a few natives with my driving. We were served this wonderful oatmeal which I have adapted to include a portion of soy. It's better than any lucky charm!

1/3 cup Irish cut oats
1/2 cup soy milk
1 tablespoon whey protein powder
2 packets Nutrasweet™

Place milk and Irish oats in a saucepan and bring to a boil. Reduce the heat and simmer for twenty minutes until soft but still liquid. It will thicken as it stands.
Blend in the sweetener.

Serves 1
per portion
Calories: 304
Protein: 20 g
Carbs: 43 g
Fat: 7 g
Sat: 2 g

lima beans with chives

2 cups frozen lima beans
Water to cover beans
1 small onion, studded with 3 whole cloves
5 whole Tellicherry black peppercorns
1 thyme sprig
1 bay leaf
1/4 cup water
1 tablespoon extra-virgin olive oil
sea salt
2 tablespoons fresh minced chives

Place the beans in a microwave safe container and add water to cover the beans, onion, peppercorns, thyme and bay leaf. Microwave on high for 5 minutes. Drain the beans, discarding the spices. Chop the onion into pieces and add to the beans.
In a large skillet, combine the beans with 1/4 cup water and cook over moderately high heat, stirring, for 2 minutes. Add the olive oil, season with salt and pepper, sprinkle with the chives and serve.

Serves 8
per portion
Calories: 60
Protein: 2 g
Carbs: 8 g
Fat: 2 g
Sat: <1 g

black beans with garlic, cilantro and cumin

Serves 4
per portion
Calories: 155
Protein: 8 g
Carbs: 24 g
Fat: 2 g
Sat: <1 g

This dish is typical of the Latin style of preparing black beans. It's quick, easy and the fragrance will make you yearn for a cabana on the beach.

15 ounces black beans, canned
2 garlic cloves
1 teaspoon ground cumin
1 teaspoon extra-virgin olive oil
1/3 cup tomato juice
3/4 teaspoon sea salt
2 tablespoons chopped cilantro

Rinse the black beans and drain. Chop the garlic.
In a nonstick skillet cook garlic and cumin in oil over moderate heat, stirring, until fragrant. Add black beans, juice, salt and cook, stirring until beans are heated through. Stir in cilantro and serve.

rosemary and lemon pinto beans

Serves 4
per portion
Calories: 96
Protein: 5 g
Carbs: 16 g
Fat: 1 g
Sat: <1 g

1 15-ounce can pinto beans, rinsed and drained
1/3 cup thinly sliced red onion
1 teaspoon extra-virgin olive oil
1 tablespoon red wine vinegar
1 teaspoon minced fresh rosemary
1 garlic clove, minced
Dash hot pepper sauce

Combine the ingredients in a bowl and toss to blend. Season to taste with salt and pepper.

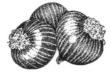

bahian black bean chili

While presenting at a conference in Rio de Janeiro, I was treated to a Brazilian dinner in the home of a friend. His wife prepared this chili which was even better the next morning for breakfast. For an extra kick, try adding sweet Spanish smoked paprika. Your family will love the samba beat it puts in your step.

Serves 8
per portion
Calories: 221
Protein: 9 g
Carbs: 38 g
Fat: 3 g
Sat: <1 g

4 teaspoons extra-virgin olive oil
1 clove garlic, minced
2 medium yellow onions, diced
1 medium poblano chili, diced
2 tablespoons cumin seed
2 tablespoons oregano
1 teaspoon cayenne pepper
1 1/2 teaspoons paprika
1 teaspoon sea salt
1/2 cup jalapeno chili, chopped with seeds
2 15-ounce cans black beans
24 ounces Muir Glen organic tomatoes, crushed
5 teaspoons soy powder
8 sprigs cilantro plus 2 tablespoons chopped
1/2 cup green onions, finely chopped
8 tablespoons white vinegar
2 medium oranges

Heat an iron skillet dry on high heat, then add the olive oil and saute the garlic, onions and poblano chili on medium heat until soft.

Add the cumin, oregano, cayenne pepper, paprika and sea salt to the mixture along with the tomatoes and chili and saute for 10 minutes on low heat.

Add the beans, soy and chopped cilantro and stir.

To serve, place the hot chili in a heated bowl, and sprinkle with some green onion. Float a tablespoon of vinegar on the top.

Cut oranges into quarters and serve alongside the chili.

red lentil and tofu curry

Serves 4
per portion
Calories: 136
Protein: 10 g
Carbs: 19 g
Fat: 3 g
Sat: <1 g

Red lentils are actually orange, but they create a creamy base when cooked. Lentils supply a hefty dose of fiber, protein, complex carbohydrate and impressive complements of iron, thiamin, niacin, phosphorus and potassium.

1 small yellow onion
1 garlic clove
1/2 inch piece of fresh gingerroot
1/2 cup red lentils, uncooked
1 teaspoon canola oil
3 1/2 cups water
1/2 cup firm tofu
1/2 teaspoon cumin seeds
1/2 teaspoon garam masala or curry powder
    (see Resources)
1/2 teaspoon sea salt
Pinch of cayenne
cilantro to garnish

Thinly slice onion and mince garlic. Peel gingerroot and mince. In a sieve, rinse lentils, removing any stones, and drain.

In a 2 quart heavy saucepan cook onion and garlic in 1 teaspoon oil over moderate heat, stirring until golden. Add gingerroot and cook, stirring, 1 minute. Add lentils and water and gently bring to a boil, uncovered, until lentils fall apart, about 20 minutes.

While lentils are boiling, rinse and drain tofu and cut into small squares.

In a heavy skillet, spray with oil and cook cumin seeds, stirring until a shade darker, about 1 minute. Add garam masala, salt, and cayenne and cook, stirring, until fragrant, 15 to 30 seconds. Stir hot spice oil into the lentils and gently stir in the tofu cubes. Let curry stand, covered, 5 minutes to allow flavors to develop. Sprinkle with cilantro and serve.

fruits and desserts

roasted peaches with cardamom

I never knew that roasting peaches could taste so good. Just inhale the fragrance as you serve them and you'll think you're lost in an orchard in Georgia.

6 ripe, firm peaches
1 tablespoon lemon juice
1 tablespoon unsalted butter
1 cinnamon stick, broken into 3 pieces
pinch of ground cloves
1 tablespoon ground cardamom
1 tablespoon grated lemon zest
3 tablespoons almond slices
1 small bunch mint leaves

Preheat oven to 400 degrees.

Dip the peaches in a pot of boiling water for 30 seconds, then place in ice water. Remove from the water and peel the skin. Quarter the peaches, removing the pits. Gently rub with lemon juice to prevent discoloration.

Melt the butter in large saucepan and add the cinnamon, cloves, cardamom and lemon zest. Cook over low heat for about 15 minutes, stirring occasionally. Add the peaches to the spicy butter, toss gently and transfer to a roasting pan. Bake for 15 minutes.

Arrange on a platter, sprinkle almonds and mint on top of the fruit.

Serves 6
per portion
Calories: 78
Protein: 1 g
Carbs: 11 g
Fat: 4 g
Sat: 1 g

white sangria splash

Serves 8
per portion
Calories: 82
Protein: 3 g
Carbs: 8 g
Fat: 2 g
Sat: 1 g

This recipe comes from the JELL-O people and makes a sophisticated dessert that's low in calories yet packed with fruit. If you use mineral water you can get your calcium too!

1 cup dry white wine
1 package (8 serving size) JELL-O brand
    lemon flavor sugar free low calorie gelatin dessert
3 cups cold club soda or mineral water
1 tablespoon lime juice
1 tablespoon orange juice
1 cup green and/or red grapes
1 cup sliced strawberries
1 cup yogurt
2 tablespoons whipping cream

Bring the wine to boil in a small saucepan. Stir boiling wine into gelatin in a medium bowl at least 2 minutes until completely dissolved. Stir in the club soda, lime juice and orange juice. Reserve one cup of the gelatin at room temperature.

Place the bowl of gelatin in a larger bowl of ice water. Let stand about 10 minutes or until thickened, stirring occasionally. If the spoon drawn through the mixture leaves definite impressions, it is ready for the next step.

Add the grapes and strawberries. Pour into three 2 cup molds or one 6 cup mold. Refrigerate about 2 hours or until set but not firm (should stick to your finger).

Stir the yogurt and whipping cream into the reserved gelatin with a wire whisk until smooth. Pour over the gelatin mold.

Refrigerate 4 hours or until firm. Unmold. Garnish as desired.

winter fruit salad

I have a lovely kumquat tree in my backyard that yields fruit nearly year round, but especially in the winter. This salad is colorful and has a great flavor.

6 kumquats, halved, seeded and coarsely chopped
2 tablespoons coarsely chopped cilantro
2 teaspoons extra-virgin olive oil
2-1/2 tablespoons fresh squeezed lemon juice
2-1/2 tablespoons coarsely chopped cilantro
1/2 teaspoon sea salt
1 large Bosc pear, peeled, cored and cut into 1/2-inch dice
1 medium cucumber, peeled,
    seeded and cut into 1/2-inch dice
1 cup coarsely chopped stemmed watercress

Serves 4
per portion
Calories: 77
Protein: 1 g
Carbs: 14 g
Fat: 3 g
Sat: <1 g

In a small bowl, combine the kumquats and cilantro with the olive oil, lemon juice and salt and let steep for 5 minutes.

In a large bowl, toss together the pear and cucumber and add the dressing and toss well. Add the watercress and toss again.

strawberries with cassis, balsamic vinegar and mint

This is an ingenious Italian dessert that presents a rich sweet and sour taste. I first enjoyed this at the La Varenne Cooking School in Paris.

1 pound strawberries
2 tablespoons creme de cassis
1 tablespoon balsamic vinegar
6 large mint leaves, cut into slices
black pepper

Serves 4
per portion
Calories: 92
Protein: 1 g
Carbs: 16 g
Fat: 1 g
Sat: 0 g

Cut the berries in half.

Toss with the creme de cassis and refrigerate, covered for one hour or more.

Just before serving, toss with the balsamic vinegar and mint. Crack fresh pepper over top.

yellow tomato, watermelon and arugula salad

Serves 4
per portion
Calories: 48
Protein: 1 g
Carbs: 6 g
Fat: 3 g
Sat: <1 g

Finally, a tomato you can pop into your mouth without fear of squishing seeds out the side. Look for these teardrop tomatoes in both red and yellow in your local farmer's market or grocery store. It's a great way to put more lycopene, a chemical that fights cancer, in your diet.

3/4 cup watermelon, cubed
2 tablespoon balsamic vinegar
2 teaspoons extra-virgin olive oil
2 ounces arugula leaves, large stems removed
3/4 pound yellow teardrop tomatoes, sliced in half

In a medium bowl, toss the watermelon cubes with one tablespoon of the vinegar and season with salt and pepper. Let stand for 5 minutes, then drain.

In a small bowl, whisk the remaining tablespoon of vinegar with the olive oil and toss with the arugula. Mix together the tomatoes, watermelon and salad and serve.

apple in dutch chocolate

Serves 1
per portion
Calories: 101
Protein: 2 g
Carbs: 25 g
Fat: <1 g
Sat: 0 g

Gillian Anderson gave this secret away. Any fruit will do, but Fuji or Gala apples seem the tastiest when dipped in this chocolate powder.

1 Fuji or Gala apple
1 package Swiss Miss™ Diet Hot Cocoa Mix
Cut apple into wedges. Do not peel.

Rip package of hot cocoa mix open. Hold in your non-dominant hand.

Carefully dip the apple wedges into the mix and enjoy!

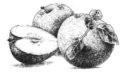

spicy fruit salad

1 16-ounce can sliced peaches
2 3-inch-long cinnamon sticks
   (use Mexican cinnamon if available)
3/4 teaspoon ground allspice
2 large navel oranges
2 large pink grapefruits
1 small pineapple
2 pints strawberries
3 kiwifruits
2 tablespoons chopped crystallized ginger

Serves 8
per portion
Calories: 106
Protein: 2 g
Carbs: 26 g
Fat: 1 g
Sat: 0 g

Drain syrup from peaches into small saucepan. Place peaches in large bowl.

Over medium-high heat, heat syrup, cinnamon, and ground allspice to boiling.

Reduce heat to low; cover and simmer 10 minutes. Set syrup mixture aside to cool while preparing fruit.

Grate peel from 1 orange; set aside. Cut peel from oranges and grapefruits.

To catch juice, hold fruit over bowl with peaches and cut sections from oranges and grapefruits between membranes; drop sections into bowl.

Cut peel and core from pineapple; cut fruit into 1 1/2-inch chunks. Add pineapple to fruit in bowl.

Pour syrup mixture over fruit in bowl. Add grated orange peel; toss.

Cover and refrigerate until ready to serve.

Just before serving, hull strawberries; cut strawberries in half if large. Cut peel from kiwifruits. Slice each kiwifruit lengthwise into 6 wedges. Toss strawberries and kiwifruits with fruit mixture. Place fruit salad in serving bowl. Sprinkle with crystallized ginger.

kir royale mold

Serves 8
per portion
Calories: 38
Protein: 2 g
Carbs: 4 g
Fat: 2 g
Sat: 1 g

2 cups boiling water
1 package (8 serving size) JELL-O brand
    Sparkling White Grape sugar free low
    calorie gelatin dessert
1 1/2 cups club soda or mineral water
2 tablespoons creme de cassis liqueur
1 tablespoon whipping cream
2 cups raspberries

Stir the boiling water into the gelatin in a large bowl at least 2 minutes until completely dissolved. Refrigerate 15 minutes.

Gently stir in the cold club soda, liqueur and whipping cream. Refrigerate for 30 minutes or until slightly thickened (the consistency of unbeaten egg whites). Gently stir for 15 seconds and add the raspberries.

Pour into a 6 cup mold and refrigerate for 4 hours or until firm. Unmold and garnish as desired.

fruit with string cheese

Serves 1
per portion
Calories: 178
Protein: 8 g
Carbs: 25 g
Fat: 7 g
Sat: 0 g

I keep small individual packages of string cheese to eat with any fruit.

1 package string cheese
1 pear

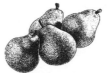

seasonings and rubs

These are recipes for seasonings that can make any simple dish a gourmet delight. I keep them on hand for grilling and they really bring out the flavor of poultry when placed under the skin.

adobo seasoning

2 tablespoons Pasilla chili powder
2 tablespoons paprika
5 teaspoons Mexican oregano
1 tablespoon ground cumin
1 tablespoon ground mustard
2 tablespoons sea salt
3/4 teaspoon cayenne pepper

Combine seasoning in a bowl. Store in a covered container.

arkansas spice rub

2 tablespoons ground cumin
1 tablespoon chili powder
1 tablespoon dry mustard
1 tablespoon coarse sea salt
1 1/2 teaspoons cayenne pepper
1 1/2 teaspoons ground cardamom
1 1/2 teaspoons ground cinnamon

Combine all in a bowl and use to rub on meats.

california bbq seasoning

I have used this seasoning combination on ribs and chicken with no complaints from any of my guests. I often place it under the skin of a turkey or chicken for extra flavor.

1 cup of kosher salt
1/2 cup garlic powder
3 tablespoons cayenne
1 tablespoon white pepper
1 tablespoon black pepper
1 teaspoon onion powder

danish rub

This spice combination is especially good on salmon if you are preparing graavlax or lox.

3 tablespoons whole coriander seeds
3 tablespoons dill seeds
3 tablespoons yellow mustard seeds
6 tablespoons whole fennel seeds
3 tablespoons sea salt
1 1/2 teaspoons Tellicherry black peppercorns

Combine all the seeds in a skillet over medium heat, shaking the pan until aromatic, about 4 minutes.

Using a spice grinder, coarsely grind seeds. Add salt and peppercorns and grind again. Keeps at room temperature in an airtight container for up to 6 months.

italian seasoning

I first enjoyed this seasoning at Tra Vigne restaurant in Napa Valley. It was served on their grilled roast chicken. You will never eat plain chicken again after tasting this.

1 cup sea salt or kosher salt
3 tablespoons Pasilla chile powder (see Resources)
2 tablespoons Ancho chile powder (see Resources)
1 tablespoon fennel
1 tablespoon cumin
1 teaspoon coriander

Grind in spice mill and store in a covered container.

tunisian seasoning

1 teaspoon sea salt
1/4 teaspoon cumin seeds
1/4 teaspoon coriander seeds
1/4 teaspoon fennel seeds
1/4 teaspoon Aleppo pepper (see Resources)
1/8 teaspoon nigella (see Resources)

Place in a spice grinder and blend. Store in an airtight container.

moroccan seasoning

1 tablespoon paprika
1 teaspoon turmeric
1/2 teaspoon cumin
1/2 teaspoon cinnamon
1/2 teaspoon ginger

Blend and use with any liquid to baste fish or poultry.

ras el hanout

This is the "top of the shop" spice mixture from Morocco. In its classic form it has 27 spices, but here is a much simpler version. You can also obtain various mixtures by direct mail (see Resources).

1 teaspoon cumin seeds
1 teaspoon ginger
1 1/2 teaspoons coriander seeds
1 1/2 teaspoons black peppercorns
    (preferably Tellicherry)
1/4 teaspoon cayenne pepper
4 whole cloves
6 allspice berries
1 1/2 teaspoons ground cinnamon
    (preferably Mexican)

Grind in a spice mill and store in an airtight jar.

reduced apple cider

Makes 2 cups
per tablespoon
Calories: 53
Protein: <1 g
Carbs: 13 g
Fat: <1 g
Sat: 0 g

This is a great base to have on hand whenever a recipe calls for honey. By reducing apple cider, you have a concentrate that works equally well as a glaze for meat, in sauces and in salad dressings. Do not use sparkling cider.

1 gallon apple cider

In a large saucepan, boil the cider over high heat until reduced to 1 quart, about 1 1/2 hours. Reduce the heat to moderate and simmer until further reduced to the consistency of maple syrup, about 45 minutes. Let the cider cool completely, then store in a tightly sealed jar in the refrigerator. It will keep indefinitely.

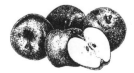

sauces, salsas and dressings

ancho-sun dried tomato pesto

This is great with pork or chicken and is easy to make. Sun dried tomatoes have a wonderful flavor and keep forever in a cool, dark place, so keep some on hand in your pantry.

4 large, dried ancho chilis, stemmed, seeded,
    torn into pieces (see Resources)
4 sun-dried tomatoes (not in oil), chopped
2/3 cup chopped roasted red peppers from a jar
2 tablespoons apple cider vinegar
1 tablespoon extra-virgin olive oil
1 tablespoon sesame seeds

Place chilis and tomatoes in a medium metal bowl and add enough boiling water to cover; let soften 20 minutes. Drain chilis and tomatoes, reserving 3/4 cup soaking liquid. Transfer chilis, tomatoes and reserved liquid to blender. Add remaining ingredients; blend until smooth. Season with salt and pepper.

Can be made 2 days ahead. Cover and chill.

Serves 12
per portion
Calories: 48
Protein: 2 g
Carbs: 7 g
Fat: 2 g
Sat: <1 g

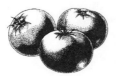

tomato and caper sauce

Serves 4
per portion
Calories: 54
Protein: 2 g
Carbs: 7 g
Fat: 3 g
Sat: <1 g

This is excellent served over fish or grilled chicken. Capers give a wonderful, piquant flavor to tomatoes so keep a jar handy in the refrigerator.

2 teaspoons extra-virgin olive oil
1 tablespoon minced, fresh garlic
2 tablespoons capers
2 cups cored and chopped fresh
    or drained canned tomatoes
Basil leaves, minced or chiffonade style
sea salt, black pepper

Heat olive oil in a medium-to-large skillet over medium heat. Add the garlic and cook until lightly colored, being careful not to burn the garlic.

Add the capers and cook for 15 seconds, then add the tomatoes and cook until thick, about 10 minutes. Season with salt and pepper.

watermelon, cantaloupe and red pepper salsa

Makes 4 cups
per cup
Calories: 59
Protein: 1 g
Carbs: 13 g
Fat: <1 g
Sat: 0 g

3/4 pound watermelon, diced
1/2 pound cantaloupe, diced
1/2 red bell pepper
1/2 small sweet onion (Vidalia, Maui, Walla Walla)
1/3 cup packed fresh cilantro sprigs
1/2 fresh jalapeno chili
2 tablespoons chopped fresh spearmint leaves
1 tablespoon fresh lime juice
sea salt

Remove rinds and seeds from the melons and cut fruit into 1/4-inch dice. Devein and deseed bell pepper and cut into 1/4-inch dice.

Finely chop onion, cilantro and jalapeno chili, including the seeds.

In a bowl, combine all the ingredients and season with sea salt.

citrus salsa

In New Zealand, my friends Helen and Richard took me to a small, local restaurant in the Wairarapa that served this salsa over fish. I even enjoy it as a salad.

1 English cucumber, seeded and diced
2 red bell peppers, seeded and diced
1 small red onion, diced
1 jalapeno chili, diced
1 tablespoon capers
2 limes, zested
2 navel oranges, zested
1 tablespoon chopped fresh mint leaves
2 tablespoons extra-virgin olive oil
sea salt

Combine the diced cucumber, pepper, onion and jalapeno chili in a non-reactive bowl. Drain the capers. Finely grate the zest from the limes and oranges and cut the citrus sections free from the membranes and cut into 1/2-inch pieces. Combine all the ingredients, toss and season with salt.

Serves 12
per portion
Calories: 47
Protein: 1 g
Carbs: 7 g
Fat: 2 g
Sat: <1 g

tarragon chive sauce

1/2 cup mayonnaise, reduced fat
1/3 cup fresh tarragon leaves
1-1/3 cup yogurt
3 tablespoons finely chopped chives
1 teaspoon lime juice
sea salt, pepper

In a food processor pulse together mayonnaise, tarragon and 1/3 cup of the yogurt until smooth. Transfer mixture to a bowl and stir in remaining cup yogurt, chives, lime juice and salt and pepper to taste.
Garnish with chives.

Makes 2 cups
per tablespoon
Calories: 37
Protein: 1 g
Carbs: 1 g
Fat: 3 g
Sat: 1 g

navy bean, garlic and tomato salsa

Makes 4 cups
per 1/3 cup
Calories: 54
Protein: 3 g
Carbs: 12 g
Fat: <1 g
Sat: 0 g

1 head garlic
1 16-ounce can navy beans
3 medium vine-ripened tomatoes (about 1-1/4 pounds)
1 small sweet onion (Vidalia, Walla Walla, Maui)
1/2 cup packed fresh basil leaves
2 tablespoons fresh lemon juice
sea salt

Preheat oven to 400 degrees.

Cut off the top of a head of garlic, wrap in foil and bake for 30 minutes. Unwrap garlic and cool. Peel skins from each clove and in a bowl mash the garlic pulp until smooth.

Rinse and drain enough beans to measure 1 cup and add to the garlic.

Cut 2 tomatoes into 1/4-inch dice and add to the beans. Quarter remaining tomato and in a blender puree until smooth. Add puree to the bean mixture.

Finely chop onion and basil and add to the bean mixture with lemon juice, tossing to combine. Season salsa with sea salt and pepper.

white wine sauce with grapes and tarragon

Serves 4
per portion
Calories: 63
Protein: 1 g
Carbs: 5 g
Fat: 2 g
Sat: <1 g

2 teaspoons extra-virgin olive oil
2 medium shallots, minced
1 tablespoon chopped fresh tarragon leaves
1/2 cup dry white wine
1 cup seedless grapes, halved lengthwise
1/2 cup fat free, reduced sodium chicken broth
sea salt, pepper

Heat pan over medium heat and add olive oil. Saute shallots until softened, about 1 minute. Add tarragon, wine and grapes; increase heat to medium-high and bring to a boil. Cook until reduced and syrupy, 4 to 5 minutes.

Add chicken broth, stirring occasionally until thickened and reduced to 3/4 cup, about 4 minutes. Adjust seasoning.

chili verde sauce

Another of Emma's great sauces from Oaxaca. Watch for tomatillos in season as they are sweeter than canned. The sticky paper wrapping around them comes off easily if you rinse them under water first. If you serve this sauce over chicken, turkey or pork, just stand back and accept the applause.

1 pound green tomatillos in the husk
1 serrano chili with seeds
2 cloves of garlic
1 bunch of cilantro
1/4 white onion, chopped
1 teaspoon of cumin whole seeds
2 teaspoons peanut oil
sea salt

Serves 12
per portion
1/3 cup
Calories: 23
Protein: 0 g
Carbs: 3 g
Fat: 1 g
Sat: 0 g

Steam tomatillos and chilis for twenty minutes. Cool.

Place the tomatillos, chilis, garlic, cilantro, onion and cumin in the blender on lowest setting. Once the initial chopping is done, blend on high.

Heat an iron skillet dry on high heat, then add the peanut oil and pour the mixture into the skillet. Immediately reduce the heat and simmer, uncovered until the desired consistency.

Season with sea salt.

raspberry vinaigrette

3/4 cup raspberry vinegar
1/3 cup chopped shallots
2 tablespoons extra-virgin olive oil
sea salt, white pepper

Serves 6
per portion
Calories: 50
Protein: <1 g
Carbs: 3 g
Fat: 5 g
Sat: 1 g

Blend vinegar and shallots in a blender or food processor. With the machine running, gradually add the oil and season with salt and pepper.

fennel-tarragon vinaigrette

Serves 8
per portion
Calories: 51
Protein: <1 g
Carbs: <1 g
Fat: 6 g
Sat: 1 g

2 tablespoons white wine vinegar
4 teaspoons chopped fresh tarragon
2 teaspoons Dijon mustard
1 teaspoon fennel seeds, crushed
3-1/3 tablespoons extra-virgin olive oil

Whisk first 4 ingredients in a medium bowl to blend. Gradually whisk in oil and season vinaigrette with salt and pepper.

jalapeno lime vinaigrette

Makes 1 cup
per tablespoon
Calories: 45
Protein: 0 g
Carbs: <1 g
Fat: 4 g
Sat: <1 g

1 2-inch fresh jalapeno chili
2/3 cup fresh lime juice
1 tablespoon rice wine vinegar
1/3 cup canola oil

In a blender combine the first three ingredients. With the motor running, add oil in a stream and blend 30 seconds or until emulsified.

yogurt, chive and dijon mustard dressing

Serves 4
per portion
Calories: 53
Protein: 2 g
Carbs: 2 g
Fat: 4 g
Sat: 1 g

1/3 cup whole milk yogurt
3 tablespoons Dijon mustard
2 tablespoons reduced-fat mayonnaise
1 bunch fresh chopped chives

In a small bowl whisk together all the dressing ingredients. Chill, covered for 1 day.

roasted pumpkin seed oil vinaigrette

I fell in love with this oil just for its radiant orange color, then discovered the wonderful flavor it imparts to greens. This type of oil tends to become bitter if heated, so it's best not to use it for cooking.

1/4 cup fresh orange juice
2 tablespoons soy sauce
1 tablespoon plus 1 teaspoon roasted pumpkin seed oil
2 teaspoons white wine vinegar
1 teaspoon minced jalapeno chili
1 garlic clove, minced
1/2 teaspoon fresh, minced ginger
sea salt, pepper

   Combine all the ingredients in a bowl and refrigerate overnight. Serve at room temperature on grilled shrimp or an avocado-tomato salad.

Serves 4
per portion
Calories: 54
Protein: 1 g
Carbs: 3 g
Fat: 5 g
Sat: <1 g

shallot vinaigrette

4 tablespoons extra-virgin olive oil
1/4 cup plus 2 tablespoons cider vinegar
2 shallots, minced
sea salt, pepper

   In a small bowl, combine all the oil, vinegar and shallots and season with taste with salt and pepper. Bring to a boil on the stove and pour over greens, such as baby spinach leaves.

Serves 8
per portion
Calories: 63
Protein: <1 g
Carbs: 1 g
Fat: 7 g
Sat: 1 g

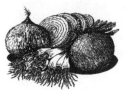

sherry-mustard dressing

Serves 6
per portion
Calories: 65
Protein: <1 g
Carbs: 1 g
Fat: 7 g
Sat: 1 g

3 tablespoons chopped shallots
2 tablespoons sherry wine vinegar
1 teaspoon Dijon mustard
3 tablespoons extra-virgin olive oil

Whisk first three ingredients together in a medium bowl to blend. Gradually whisk in oil and season with sea salt and pepper to taste.

chipotle dressing

Serves 6
per portion
Calories: 67
Protein: <1 g
Carbs: 1 g
Fat: 7 g
Sat: 1 g

1/4 cup fresh orange juice
1 tablespoon finely chopped canned chipotle chilis
1/4 teaspoon ground cinnamon, preferably Mexican
1 teaspoon ground cumin
3 tablespoons extra-virgin olive oil

Whisk the first four ingredients together in a small bowl. Add the oil and whisk until blended.

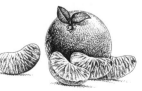

soyamaise

Real mayonnaise is made with soy oil but this version works nicely as a salad dressing, dip or sauce.

1/4 cup lemon juice
1/4 cup canola oil
4 teaspoons soy sauce
1/2 teaspoon sea salt
1/4 cup yellow onions, chopped
4 green onions, finely chopped
2 cloves garlic
1/3 cup chopped parsley
1/2 teaspoon curry powder
14 ounces tofu, drained and dried

   Place all the ingredients in a blender except the tofu and process.
   Add the tofu and blend until smooth. Refrigerate overnight.
   Makes 2 1/2 cups or 32 tablespoons.

per tablespoon
Calories: 38
Protein: 2 g
Carbs: 1 g
Fat: 3 g
Sat: 0 g

soyamaise for vegetables

1/4 cup lemon juice
1/4 cup canola oil
1 tablespoon dijon mustard
1 sprig fresh dill
1/2 teaspoon sea salt
14 ounces tofu, drained and dried

   Place all the ingredients in a blender except the tofu and process.
   Add the tofu and blend until smooth. Refrigerate overnight.

per tablespoon
Calories: 36
Protein: 2 g
Carbs: 1 g
Fat: 3 g
Sat: 0 g

dips, drinks and dairy

carlos and charlie's tuna dip

Serves 10
per portion
(3 tablespoons)
Calories: 69
Protein: 10 g
Carbs: 0 g
Fat: 3 g
Sat: 1 g

This is an updated version of an old recipe from Carlos N' Charlie's, a celebrity hangout on the Sunset Strip in Hollywood. Serve with fresh vegetables or scoop it into romaine lettuce leaves.

1 12 1/2 ounce can tuna, drained
2 jalapeno chilis, seeded and stemmed
1 (1 inch) piece green onion (green part only)
1 (1 inch) piece celery
1/4 cup light mayonnaise
sea salt, pepper
4 leaves cilantro, chopped

Blend tuna, jalapenos, green onion and celery in a food processor or blender (do not puree). Blend in mayonnaise and seasoning. Blend to desired consistency and sprinkle with cilantro.

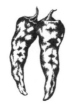

grilled eggplant dip

This recipe needs to be prepared a day ahead of time, so I often make it for weekend get-togethers with my friends. Serve it in a hollowed-out eggplant for a special effect.

Makes 3 cups
per 1/4 cup
Calories: 62
Protein: 1 g
Carbs: 6 g
Fat: 4 g
Sat: <1 g

4 pounds medium eggplants
1 small red onion
2 large garlic cloves
2/3 cup packed fresh flat-leafed parsley leaves
2-2/3 tablespoons extra-virgin olive oil
3 tablespoons white-wine vinegar
2 tablespoons reduced-fat mayonnaise

Prepare grill.

Pierce eggplants in several places with a fork and grill on a rack set 5 to 6 inches over glowing coals, turning them occasionally, until very soft, 30 to 40 minutes. (If you don't want to prepare a grill, broil them about 6 inches from a preheated broiler for 30 to 40 minutes. The smoky flavor will be missing.)

Transfer eggplants to a colander and when cool enough to handle, quarter lengthwise. Remove as many seeds as possible. Scrape the flesh into a large sieve set over a bowl, discarding the skin. Drain eggplant, covered and chilled, 1 day. Discard any juices from the eggplant.

Mince onion and garlic and finely chop parsley. In a food processor pulse eggplant with onion, garlic, parsley and remaining ingredients until coarsely pureed. Transfer spread to a bowl and season with salt and pepper. Chill dip, covered at least 3 hours.

yogurt and nuts

This is another quick, easy snack to use.

Serves 1
per portion
Calories: 161
Protein: 13 g
Carbs: 17 g
Fat: 5 g
Sat: 2 g

1 cup low-fat yogurt
1 teaspoon slivered almonds

white bean dip with garlic, lemon and basil

Serves 4
per portion
(1/3 cup)
Calories: 52
Protein: 3 g
Carbs: 8 g
Fat: 1 g
Sat: 0 g

This is a great dip to keep on hand for snacks. It seems I never make enough.

4 cups white beans, soaked and cooked if dried,
    or straight from can (reserve any liquid)
1/3 cup coarsely chopped fresh basil or parsley leaves
1/4 cup lemon juice
1 tablespoon extra-virgin olive oil
2 large garlic cloves, crushed

    Drain beans. Combine beans, basil, lemon juice, oil, and garlic in the bowl of a food processor. Process until smooth, adding reserved liquid tablespoon by tablespoon, as necessary. Add salt and pepper to taste. Refrigerate at least 1 hour.
    Serve with crisp vegetables like peppers, celery, broccoli, daikon.

white bean hummus

Makes 3 cups
per tablespoon
Calories: 25
Protein: 1 g
Carbs: 4 g
Fat: 1 g
Sat: <1 g

This is a very low calorie version of a hummus without the tahini. Serve it sprinkled with Aleppo pepper for color and a unique, smoky flavor.

2 15-ounce cans navy beans
6 garlic cloves
2 tablespoons extra-virgin olive oil
1 teaspoon ground cumin
1/2 teaspoon ground coriander seeds
1/4 teaspoon salt
Pinch of cayenne

    Rinse and drain beans. To a food processor with the motor running, drop garlic through the tube and blend until minced. Add beans and remaining ingredients and blend until smooth. Transfer to a serving bowl and chill, covered for 1 day. Just before serving sprinkle Aleppo pepper on top.

fourth of july cottage cheese

There is nothing faster than cottage cheese and fruit when you need to get out the door in a hurry. Berries lend a festive reminder of this holiday celebration, but don't substitute nonfat cottage cheese, as the fructose in the fruit will act like 3 tablespoons of corn syrup in your body.

1 cup 2% cottage cheese
1/4 cup blueberries
1/4 cup raspberries
1/4 cup strawberries

Serves 1
per portion
Calories: 227
Protein: 32 g
Carbs: 20 g
Fat: 5 g
Sat: 3 g

black currant iced tea with cinnamon and ginger

I love iced teas and this one is especially pretty when served in a frosted glass with a little cinnamon stick.

6 cups water
12 wild black currant herbal tea bags
2 3-inch long cinnamon sticks, broken in half
1 tablespoon (packed) minced, peeled fresh ginger
Nutrasweet™

Serves 8
per portion
Calories: 0
Protein: 0 g
Carbs: 0 g
Fat: 0 g
Sat: 0 g

Bring 6 cups of water to boil in a large saucepan. Add tea bags, broken cinnamon sticks and fresh ginger. Remove from the heat; cover and steep 10 minutes. Chill until cold. Strain tea mixture into pitcher and sweeten with Nutrasweet™. Serve in frosted glasses with ice and garnish with cinnamon sticks.

orangeade

---

6 cups fresh orange juice
4 1/2 cups chilled seltzer or club soda

In a large pitcher stir together juice and seltzer or club soda and garnish with orange slices. Serve in tall glasses half-filled with ice.

Makes 10 cups
per cup
Calories: 67
Protein: 1 g
Carbs: 16 g
Fat: <1 g
Sat: 0 g

sparkling berry lemonade

Serves 6
1 cup serving
Calories: 35
Protein: 1 g
Carbs: 9 g
Fat: <1 g
Sat: 0 g

Use whatever berries are in season for this delicious, cooling drink.

3 cups quartered fresh berries (strawberries,
        blueberries, blackberries, raspberries)
12 ounces fresh squeezed lemon juice
3 cups sparkling water, chilled
6 packets Nutrasweet™

Combine strawberries and lemon juice in a blender and process until smooth.

Add sparkling water and Nutrasweet; pour over ice.

herbed tomato juice

Serves 10
per portion
Calories: 37
Protein: 1 g
Carbs: 6 g
Fat: 1 g
Sat: <1 g

When tomatoes are in season, I love to make this liquified version of gazpacho and serve it in individual small, iced glass candle holders.

1 1/2 pounds ripe tomatoes, quartered
1 tablespoon extra-virgin olive oil
1 tablespoon plus 1 teaspoon red wine vinegar
2 teaspoons thyme leaves
2 teaspoons coarsely chopped tarragon
1 small garlic clove, minced
1 1/2 teaspoons sherry vinegar
Pinch of cayenne pepper
sea salt, white pepper

In a food processor combine the tomatoes, olive oil, red wine vinegar, thyme tarragon, garlic, sherry vinegar and cayenne and process until smooth. Season lightly with salt and black pepper. Transfer the puree to a bowl and refrigerate for at least 1 hour and up to 1 day.

Just before serving, strain the tomato juice through a fine sieve, pressing on the tomatoes. Season again with salt and pepper. Whisk until frothy, then pour into small cups and serve.

sassy rhubarb mint coolers

From April to June, the sassy stalks of rhubarb wave at me from the produce section, inviting me to drink in their luscious color. Long considered a spring tonic for its medicinal properties, rhubarb is really a vegetable that is painfully tart. Try this cooler topped with a jaunty hat of mint for a real change!

Serves 5
per portion
Calories: 19
Protein: 1 g
Carbs: 4 g
Fat: 0 g
Sat: 0 g

1 pound trimmed rhubarb
1 teaspoon anise seeds
5 cups water
1/4 cup packed fresh mint leaves
Nutrasweet™

Cut rhubarb into 1/2-inch pieces and in a saucepan bring to a boil with water, anise and mint leaves. Simmer mixture, stirring occasionally, 15 minutes (rhubarb will disintegrate) and cool 15 minutes. Pour mixture through a fine sieve into a pitcher, pressing hard on solids. Chill mixture, covered, until cold, about 3 hours. Add Nutrasweet™ to taste only when thoroughly chilled.

Serve coolers over ice in glasses garnished with mint sprigs.

smoky "virgin" mary

Be sure and use a vegetable or tomato juice that doesn't have any added corn syrup.

---

3 cups vegetable juice
2 tablespoons fresh lemon juice
1 tablespoon minced fresh cilantro
1 tablespoon Worcestershire sauce
1 teaspoon finely minced, seeded, canned chipotle chilies
1 teaspoon ground cumin
6 stalks celery with leafy tops for garnish

Serves 6
per portion
Calories: 26
Protein: 1 g
Carbs: 6 g
Fat: 0 g
Sat: 0 g

Mix everything but the celery in a pitcher and chill until cold, at least 2 hours or overnight.

Fill 6 tall glasses with ice and pour mixture over it. Garnish with the celery stalks.

chapter five

investing in your
health with exercise

I'll admit right now I'm not an exercise expert. I
don't like to sweat, and I'm really not good at it! Even
mentioning the "E" word can make me break out in a
rash. I've been known to turn bright red, feel like a
furnace and get a heart rate that rivals the hammering of
a fire alarm just passing a gym. Let's face it – I belong
to the school of thought that if God had wanted women
to exercise, He would have strewn the floor with
diamonds. Only about 38% of women over the age of
19 exercise regularly, and only half of middle-aged
women engage in any regular recreational exercise.[166,167]
The benefits of exercise are well known: it improves
circulation, strengthens bones, lowers blood pressure,
cholesterol and can be key in controlling your weight.
So why are less than 25% of women following the
National Institutes of Health's recommended guidelines
for light to moderate exercise for at least 30 minutes a
day, 6 days a week?

I'll be up front with you. I HATE EXERCISING,
but I've come to realize it is a necessary evil in life, like
mammograms. I get no high when I work out or feel
that rush of something that's supposed to make you feel
great. Never did, even when I danced. Instead exercising
is all work, not pleasure for me and that's a problem in
keeping me motivated. In addition, many forms of
exercise aren't really safe or suitable for those of us who
are exercise virgins. I have a graveyard of exercise
products buried under my bed that promised to tone
and condition my body in just a few minutes a day. But
then, you're talking to a woman who still believes the
weight on her drivers license is valid. So what made me

change my mind?

The more you exercise, especially if you participate in intensive physical activity, the stronger your bones and the less belly fat you retain.[168,169] Exercise counteracts the decline in our ability to burn fat, especially when our metabolism moves slower than the 405 freeway at rush hour.[170] When you vigorously exercise, such as running or playing several games of tennis, you can significantly lower the amount of dangerous intra-abdominal fat you carry.[171,172] But here's the catch—women who are overweight are the least likely to exercise vigorously, and even moderate physical activity has little or no effect on weight control or cholesterol levels in women.[173]

Say what?? The facts are clear: men, unlike women can raise the good cholesterol (HDL) and lose that Buddha Belly simply by dieting, while women require vigorous exercise in addition to calorie restriction to produce the same effects.[21] Men simply have more muscle mass, which translates into a higher resting metabolic rate.[174] To make matters worse, it doesn't make any difference if a man just barely exercises. He gets the same health benefits regardless of the degree of intensity. Not so for women.[175]

The gods must be having a good laugh at women because how else could you explain this cruel inequity? I searched diligently for contradicting evidence, any scrap of research that could prove women can lose and maintain weight loss without exercise – and that is when I experienced my own epiphany about exercising. Like "red shirting" in college, I had been given a pass in the exercise game during my early years. Shamelessly, I stood on the sidelines cheering all those other women who, like me, broke a sweat just getting their nails done. But now it was payback time and I was determined to start winning the game of weight control.

I started out by picking up fitness magazines and reading how other people conquered their aversions to exercise. Then I made a list of all the reasons I wanted to be healthy for the next twenty five years and hung it on the fridge. I itemized all the things I hated about exercise then listed ways to compensate for each one. It turned out I really had only a few objections to the Big E – sweating, boredom and pain. Then I looked at my exercise options.

run larrian run

A patient once told me she was fine until one day she ran BAM, right into menopause. I know how she feels. I have never been a fan of running. I don't see the point. Anthropologically, why would you run for hours, like in a marathon? Running is for catching something, maybe food or fleeing danger. Our pelvis, unlike a man's, was not built to withstand the bouncing tension on the pelvic floor which can lead to nerve damage. Sure the outfits are cute but I don't look good in a sweatband. Since running long distance may or may not prevent estrogen-deficient bone loss in dieting women, why do it?[176,177]

Aerobic exercise, which is any kind of sustained low intensity activity like walking, swimming, jogging or rope jumping, lowers your insulin response and helps to keep your blood sugar in line.[178] While some women find running a form of meditation in motion and feel their best if they run, I found it boring and painful. Besides, I wanted not only to improve my stamina but get a great shape. However, I passed on running for another reason and that was the risk of injury occurring to my knees.[179]

The normal anterior cruciate ligament (ACL) is critical for keeping your knee joint stable and aligned. Rupture of this ligament can be devastating as your knee becomes like a rocking horse with any motion, further injuring the meniscus, or gel pad in the joint which can lead to arthritis. Injuries to the ACL are four to eight times higher in women than men, especially during ovulation.[180] Estrogen, particularly 17 beta-estradiol, reduces collagen synthesis and weakens the ligament, making it more susceptible to injury.[181] Since women live longer than men but spend more years disabled, I wanted to avoid any method of exercise that ran an increased risk of injury. This is not to take anything away from women who enjoy running.

Remember, the key to sticking with any program is making it less work and more play. Do a risk/benefit analysis. Just be sure the enjoyment and benefits you receive from any exercise option are more than the relative risk of injury.

Treadmilling seemed a more logical way to avoid the chance of injury and still improve my cardiovascular system. A word of advice: don't purchase a unit with a motor rated less than 2 horsepower or the belt won't move smoothly and you can increase your risk of injury. Always start out with a slow warmup and then hit your stride. "Milling" is a much better weight-bearing exercise for preventing osteoporosis than a stationary bike. Besides, you can't skip on a bike.

No room for a treadmill? Purchase a beaded jump rope. This type of rope is a little more weighted and balanced than a cloth, nylon or leather rope. To choose the right size, just stand with one foot on the middle of the rope and the ends of the handles should reach and barely touch your armpits. In just a few minutes of jumping in place, you can turn on your fat burning metabolism, build bones and improve your coordination.

bent on riding

I don't like riding a bike. In fact, you could say I am "biking impaired" when it comes to handling anything with two wheels. But that all changed when I tried a "bent" or recumbent bike. It's the most fun I've ever had in a horizontal position. Okay, so I'm lying. With an estimated 15,000 recumbents sold in 1998 alone, these bikes are becoming a serious mainstream alternative for women who want a comfortable, knee-safe mode of transportation. Because you pedal in a recumbent position, it's ideal for people with short little arms and legs. Think of it as taking a spin on a Barcalounger but without the dorky looks.

What makes the ride so great? The special can-tilevered fork on the loadbearing rear wheel acts as a shock absorber and the seat cushion is padded with a great back support. You can pedal longer without tiring, which helps you to burn more fat. Your butt will shape up too because bents do less for your quads and more for your hamstrings and glutes. As for other body parts, cycling in the recumbent position lets you bear less weight on your wrists, knees, shoulders and neck.

If you're like me, crashing can be a hazard to one's health. The good news? You run into objects feet first. It only took me ten minutes to learn how to ride the new BikeE CT, making it the hands-down winner for biking virgins. Oh, and did I mention it's really a hunk magnet? Oh yeah! With a shape like a low rider, men will be begging you to let them try it. Just ignore the whimpering.

resisting change

Working with weights or resistance training overcame many of my objections to exercise. I didn't have to sweat to get the benefits of stronger bones and muscles; it wasn't really painful and it was only moderately boring. But there are different ways to achieve resistance and with them come differences in the shape your body develops.

Lifting weights has been the standard of resistance training. You can see the results from strength training in less than three months.[182,183] A word of caution: It's safest to start with a trainer in order to prevent injury. Don't use heavy weights unless you want to look like Arnold! Instead, very light weights and a high number of repetitions will give you the tiny biceps that can lift groceries or children. If you are looking for flexibility, weights are not the answer as they tighten your muscles, instead of stretch them.

pilates®

This form of resistance training has seen a new resurgence as women are looking for a long, lean look to their bodies. Developed as a rehabilitation program for injured soldiers during World War I, Pilates® emphasizes flexibility along with strength. When combined with controlled breathing, it offers a great workout. By isolating certain muscle groups, no unnecessary energy is expended and weak muscles are strengthened as bulky muscles become elongated. It's really a form of "dancing on your back" with smooth gliding motions.

The secret to Pilates® is learning posture and how to keep your abdominals taut while moving your arms and legs. It requires mental focus, as these exercises engage the whole body and mind, challenging you to concentrate on body alignment and control. It's truly a way of bringing conciousness to your muscles.

I have faithfully done this exercise program for two years, which tells you it is neither boring, sweaty nor painful. However, it is expensive and requires special equipment. You really need to do it with an instructor if you want to achieve the full benefit of this program. Pilates® is not a replacement for cardio conditioning as it is really anaerobic exercising. There are floor exercises which you can follow from several books.

yoga

Yoga offers much of the same benefits as Pilates® without requiring any equipment. There are four key exercises that will teach you the ABC's of yoga. The first one is called the Mountain pose. You literally stand like a mountain, stretching your fingers downward while feeling like a string has been drawn through the top of your head, pulling your spine upwards. This positions raises awareness of how you stand and improves your posture. The second position is the Tree pose. I think of it as standing like a stork on one foot with your other foot planted firmly against your thigh while raising your arms above your head. Balance is the key here. Just don't try this one when your dog decides to run laps around the room. The third position involves sitting on the floor with your legs and toes extended while drawing in your abdomen. This is a quiet, meditative type of position. Finally, you can sit on your heels while breathing in slowly for 2 to 3 minutes in order to connect and center yourself.

The deep breathing of yoga, combined with its stretching, is an excellent way to begin any exercise plan. The goal of exercising is to increase the exchange of oxygen by every cell in your body. Certain forms of yoga emphasize breathing in specific patterns, which can be helpful in mantaining the shape of a goddess. There are numerous videos and books on this technique which can help to limber you up for that position on page 28 of the Kama Sutra.

endurance is the key

If your goal is to firm, tone or reduce, you want to concentrate on developing good muscle endurance. That means you can hit a golf ball 200 yards on the first hole and 200 yards on the eighteenth hole four hours later. Low glycemic index carbs can do the trick because they result in higher concentrations of fuels towards the end of your exercise program when you need them most.[184] So don't rush to eat that high sugar energy bar before playing tennis. You'll only be giving your opponent the advantage. Munch on some broccoli or cottage cheese instead and stay cool to the finish.

the secret to my success

I really wish I could tell you I went to bed and woke up refreshed and ten pounds thinner, but that would only be "in my dreams." I selected a program of cross training using Pilates® two days a week, biking on my recumbent and walking on a treadmill twice a week which I conveniently placed under a ceiling fan and smack dab in front of a TV with a remote control. In this way I could stay cool and stave off boredom by watching my favorite movies or comedy shows.

You can lose weight and fat without compromising your muscle strength if you do strength training three days a week and walk two more days.[185] If you only use The Goddess Diet, you'll miss the opportunity to increase your muscle mass and its ability to burn fat.[186] In short, you'll be flying on low octane instead of jet fuel. Don't have enough time to exercise? Even short bursts of brief intense exercise can lower your sugar and insulin levels.[187] Try breaking your exercise into 10 minute segments. Come on...you can do anything for ten minutes! Take the stairs, walk to the book store or just around the block. Seize the moment and get on the treadmill while watching the news. Flexibility is the key to making exercise work for you. Treat each day like a menu – mix and match and you get a full course. As I stated, I am no exercise expert, but you will find lots of resources to explore in Appendix A to help you find an exercise program that works for you. High blood pressure is a killer but regular moderate exercise, such as walking, can significantly lower your risk of a stroke.[188] It can also nudge a sluggish gallbladder into action.[189] So don't just choose one type of exercise – mix it up and your body will thank you. And remember all those ballet and gymnastic classes your mom forced you to take? Exercising during puberty is an opportune time to increase bone density that can last into your "Golden Years" by reducing the risk of fractures after menopause.[190] This only proves mothers really DO know what's best!

Estrogen, when combined with The Goddess Diet and treadmilling, can give women who experience premature ovarian failure the same benefits as intensive exercise because the combination enhances your ability to send growth hormone levels shooting up. Now you can really burn the fat hiding deep inside your stomach.[191,192] Even strength training results in stronger bones with the assistance of estrogen.[193] Again, micro managing your hormones is important, so work with your physician to modify your dosage to suit the lowest level possible that will still give you heart, brain and bone protection.

After just three months of following The Goddess Diet Plan of mini meals and exercising, I had lost enough weight and inches to stand in the far corner of my closet looking at clothes I hadn't worn in 10 years. Suddenly, sleeves were waving furiously at me and I swore I heard cries of "Pick Me... Pick Me...I haven't been out in years! Who looks best on you baby?" But then again, maybe it was the hot sauce talking.

chapter six

why stress can make you fat

You're patiently waiting for a parking spot in a crowded shopping mall when a rogue automobile comes tearing down the aisle, swinging right into your slot. You hit the horn, start screaming and vow to flatten two tires on that sucker once you find ANOTHER spot! At that very moment you are getting fat!

Stress, especially chronic stress taxes your heart, scrambles your brain and sabotages your immune system from working like the national guard to protect your body against infection and cancer. But more importantly, even stressful thoughts can deprive your tissue of oxygen and the necessary chemicals to keep your hormones in balance.

to fight or flee: that is the question

Just imagine you're a gazelle frolicking on the Serengeti plains of Africa. Life is good and you don't have a care in the world. That is, until a lion shows up. Suddenly your heart takes the elevator to the top floor along with your blood pressure and you pass on being the blue plate special for the day and run like hell. During those few moments, your brain faxed your adrenals to squeeze out cortisol, norepinephrine and adrenaline or epinephrine to give you the energy for this life-or-death emergency. Once you are safe, your body "stands down," and resumes its normal function. Or at least that's how our bodies were designed.

Unfortunately, in our high stress society, we put ourselves through disaster training several times a day, which triggers these hormones to grab high-octane fat and quick burning glucose for energy to supply our brain, heart and muscles. And with that comes the necessity to store more fat. There's no question that cortisol increases fat deposition in one place, the worst place of all...the belly.

stress can break your heart

Women are the more fragile sex when it comes to their ability to handle stress, especially mental stress. While performing three mental stress tasks, womens' brains were studied by nuclear scanning while measurements were taken of their blood pressure. Postmenopausal women have significantly greater blood pressure reactivity than men or premenopausal women when under mental stress.[194] This is NOT a good thing. The presence of mental stress reduces the blood supply to the heart at lower heart rates than during exercise, giving a new meaning to the word "stress testing."[195] When researchers studied women who were stressed out in their day to day lives, or who felt tense, frustrated, sad and lonely, they were twice as likely to risk a heart attack in the following hour![196] If that wasn't enough, a ten year study of women who swallowed their anger but maintained a hostile attitude had higher plaque formation in their carotid arteries and could stroke out than women who expressed themselves and got on with life.[197] Despite the decrease in coronary heart disease (CHD) mortality in the US in the past 30 years, CHD kills nearly 500,000 American women each year, with African American women having a higher prevalence of CHD risk factors and a higher death rate at a younger age than white women.[198]

putting your ovaries in a twist

Stress packs a whollop throughout your whole body and can affect your ability to ovulate, a precious commodity. By firing up your sympathetic nerve pathways, the celiac plexus, a major switching station behind the stomach, stocks up on norepinephrine and signals the ovaries to release the same neural transmitter.

We put ourselves through disaster training several times a day

This accompanies an increase in testosterone and estradiol, causing precystic follicles to develop with a drop in ovulation.[199] Before you realize it, you've created a cyst, which can cause pain in your side and make you feel like weeping. When sheep are faced with a barking dog (audiovisual stress) or insulin-induced hypoglycemia (metabolic stress) they produce acute rises in adrenocortical hormone (ACTH), cortisol, epinephrine and norepinephrine which can only be turned off by high doses of estrogen.[200] If you have lowering estrogen levels, you simply don't have enough estrogen reserve to combat your stress response hormonally. And if you spend sleepless nights worrying about things, you might as well be counting pounds instead of sheep.

sick and tired

Long term stress not only causes weight gain but it does a number on your immune system. You become susceptible to colds and flus and feel just plain tired. Wounds take longer to heal because cortisol prevents the normal buildup of killer white cells in the body. Even just taking a test can stress you out and make you sick. Dental students were given wounds to the roof of their mouths three days before their final exam and again during summer vacation (does this give you an idea of what professors think of their students?). Not surprisingly, the wounds took 40% longer to heal during the test time because of a 70% decline in the production of a particular type of white blood cell messenger RNA.[201] This same response was found in caretakers of Alzheimer patients, proving that psychological stress can make you a target for illness.[202]

It takes estrogen to combat stress

who am I? where am I?

If you've ever spent hours looking for your keys, or that credit card bill that was due tomorrow, you may be experiencing some memory loss due to stress. Glucocorticoids, the adrenal steroid hormones secreted during stress, can damage the hippocampus or memory center of your brain by depriving the tissue of energy producing glucose.[203] It only takes 4 hours of stress to uncouple the neurons in your brain thanks to the plentiful receptors for corticosterone, the stress hormone in the hippocampus. This can affect your learning ability and may even cause brain cancer.[204] Repeated stress causes brain cells to shrink and can permanently damage nerve cells.[205] A recent study at McGill University in Quebec found that older people with high cortisol levels had smaller hippocampi and showed greater memory loss than their less-stressed peers. Women especially are more vulnerable to stress-induced memory loss than men. Stress hormones block the pituitary's ability to send signals to the ovary to ovulate and these same hormones make your ovaries less responsive. The net result is estrogen, leutenizing and follicle stimulating hormones are suppressed. Without estrogen, there is no control over damage from corticosterone in the brain.[206] No wonder you seem to be having a "senior moment" about those car keys.

Sleep deprivation can lower your metabolism

fattening up your sleep cycle can trim your weight

You open your left eye and peek at the clock. It's 2 AM and you can't get back to sleep, so you turn on the TV just to hear the test pattern play white noise in the background. You feel unhappy and depressed – sort of out of sync with your life. Unfortunately, disturbances in your ability to sleep can cause you to gain weight.

Serotonin, that feel good hormone, is a precursor to melatonin, which is produced by the pineal gland in the brain, a pea size organ behind the hypothalamus. The role of melatonin is to help regulate your sleep, but women can have low levels due to changes in their hormone status.[207] Melatonin has other roles, and one of them is the regulation of glucose by the central nervous system in a non-insulin dependent manner.[208] When you sleep, melatonin levels go up in response to darkness and go down when your eyes are exposed to light. But if you are unable to stay asleep long enough, you disturb the glucose levels in your blood that keep your brain fed during the night.[209] Your body rhythm gets out of whack and this causes less growth hormone to be produced.

Remember, growth hormone and estrogen mobilize fat in the body, while cortisol and insulin store fat. Growth hormone (GH) peaks during sleep just before you start to dream, so if you don't get several episodes of rapid eye movement sleep (REM) in a night, you can't produce sufficient GH and melatonin to keep blood glucose levels in check. But that's not all the problem sleep deprivation can have on our health. It can lower your metabolism by dropping thyroid hormone levels, increase your blood sugar and acclerate metabolic aging.[210] In short, you get fat.

Just in case you thought taking melatonin was the answer to burning the midnight oil – think again. Melatonin increases the production of somatostatin, a hormone that turns off glucagon and growth hormone production. It takes the rhythm of darkness and light in a 24 hour period to turn it back on. Sleep deprivation can lower your metabolism. Several studies have looked at obesity and sleep disturbances and found that both depression and sleep alterations were signs of insulin resistance.[211-213] In particular, abdominal weight gain was confirmed by an increased waist-hip ratio due to high levels of cortisol directing fat storage to the abdomen instead of the thighs.[214] Tossing and turning all night consistently inhibits the ability of the body to produce GH-releasing hormone, which signals the body to produce GH and increases the amount of insulin-like growth factor-I. This is all corrected when sleep is restored.[215]

Tossing and turning can make you fat

don't hold your breath

Another important medical problem, sleep apnea or breath holding, can happen when you don't get enough sleep. Studies have shown a strong link between a Buddha Belly and sleep apnea. It seems sleep is a very active metabolic time for us, and if we don't get enough oxygen during the night we can gain weight or prevent the loss of weight by reducing the production of growth hormone and estrogen. This changes your energy balance and insulin sensitivity creating a change in your brain's response to serotonin.[216] In a study of the relationship between lowered sympathetic nerve activity and obesity, researchers found that we become more sensitive to essential fatty acids when our serotonin levels drop and that makes you not only fat but depressed.[217,218]

stress busters

So, now that you realize how destructive stress can be in your life, what are you going to do about it? Here is what I found helpful:

- **Laugh.** It may sound silly, but laughter not only supplies oxygen to your body, it creates movement. I am personally addicted to episodes of "Absolutely Fabulous" but I have been known to slip an occasional "Fawlty Towers" cassette into my player and roll on the floor in hysterics.

- **Sing.** The benefits of singing are numerous, especially if you learn to sing from your diaphragm (the part beneath your rib cage... not the one in your drawer!!) I especially recommend doing it in a foreign language so as to eliminate the embarrassment of not remembering the words.

- **Dance.** There is nothing more stress relieving than an attack of "Happy Feet." It doesn't matter what style you choose, just move and breathe and feel the rhythm of the music.

- **Walk.** Take 15 minutes a day to soak in the sunshine. Not only will you improve your mood but it can help you lose weight by adjusting your melatonin cycle and making you more responsive to insulin.[219]

- **Pose.** Just making yourself be still can help blow off steam. Yoga or meditation are ways to lower the stress hormones. For others, running helps them meditate in motion. If you're feeling stressed, assume the balance pose or T posture. Begin by standing comfortably, arms at your sides, and slowly fold forward from the hips. Extend your arms past your ears and bring your torso parallel to the ground. Simultaneously extend your left leg straight behind you. Breathe deeply and aim for stillness. Gently come back to your standing position and switch sides.

• **Primp.** Pamper yourself. Remember, you're a goddess and worth every cent you earn or spend. Take a bubble bath, a steam shower or soak in a hot tub filled with flower petals.

• **Sleep.** Get to bed by 9:00 PM. Melatonin levels start to rise around 9:30 so pay attention to how much light you are exposed to in a 24 hour period. At least 9 hours of sleep are required by your body to reset your biological clock and improve your insulin sensitivity.

• **Inhale.** Pay attention to aromas. Cleopatra soaked the sails of her ship in fragrant oils to announce her approach to Rome. Try relaxing oils of ylang ylang, bergamot, tuberose, motia or orange soaked on a cotton ball. Inhaling a fragrance can stir pleasing memories which cause endorphins, the body's natural pain killers, to be released. Burn a candle or put a diffuser in your room. Just a few whiffs of lavender oil can lull you to sleep.

• **Pray.** Prayer-walking, also known as "walking meditation" provides an easy way to be active and relieve stress. It can be a meandering saunter down a garden path or a brisk march around a track. The point is to walk with prayerful intentions realizing that your journey is an interior one.

Post inspirational quotes around your work area and be thankful for being alive. There's more to life than you'll ever realize and every day brings new chances to share.

chapter seven

nutritional support: a helping hand

If you follow the concepts of The Goddess Diet, you should realize you are improving your vitamin balance by eating nutritionally dense foods. However, since you will be eliminating many of the "fortified" grains and starches until you reach a healthy weight, the addition of selected nutritional supplements is like buying collision insurance. So let's go over what nutrients may behave like an airbag in your diet.

- **Calcium** is essential for women of all ages to promote healthy bones and lower high blood pressure. It can reduce the risk of cancer of the colon, strokes and even kidney stones. In a study of dietary fat and calcium intakes, postmenopausal women ate more than the recommended amount of dietary fat while ignoring foods high in calcium.[220] Even the dietary intake of calcium in Chinese women was below the recommended daily allowance, putting them at risk for osteoporotic fractures.[221] Good sources are all dairy products except butter, lentils, most dark leafy greens and the soft bones of sardines. The easiest way to consume calcium is in mineral water. Supplementation with 800mg/d may prevent osteoporosis in post-menopausal women when given along with Vitamin D.[222] If you are concerned about bone loss, use a calcium supplement with bicarbonate as the anion or negative charged molecule. You actually strengthen and increase the amount of bone production in your body by alkalinizing your system.[223] I take 750mg of calcium carbonate a day.

• **Folic acid,** one of the B vitamins, lowers blood levels of homocysteine, a risk factor for atherosclerotic disease. A simple deficiency of this vitamin can trigger 30 to 40% of the heart attacks and strokes suffered in America.[224] In a study of folate intake and its effect on homocysteine levels, researchers found the current RDA of 180 microg/d failed to maintain low levels of this amino acid and recommended an intake of 516 microg/d to decrease the levels of homocysteine in postmenopausal women.[225] Folic acid can also protect against cancer by altering DNA changes in your white blood cells. Good sources for folate are liver, nuts, lentils, spinach and other dark leafy greens, oranges and avocados. For the best availability of folate, choose fresh produce from a Farmer's market or the organic section of your grocery store.

• **Beta carotene,** a precursor of Vitamin A, is believed to reduce the risk of certain types of cancer. It's water soluble, which means if you take too much you'll wind up nourishing your toilet bowl. Food sources such as dark orange fruits and vegetables, like winter squash, pack an amazing amount of beta carotene into a single serving. As several foods containing beta carotene are high glycemic foods, I supplement my diet with 5000 iu a day.

• **Vitamin E** or d-alpha tocopherol is a powerful antioxidant which acts like a bug zapper to protect the first line of defense of any cell — its membrane. Vitamin E, which is fat soluble, helps keep the good cholesterol high (HDL) while lowering the bad cho-lesterol (LDL) and can reduce the swelling from arthritis while slowing down the development of cataracts. Good sources are peanut butter, liver, leafy greens, soybeans and nuts. Dosages above 800iu may cause hypertension. As freezing of vegetables destroys the activity of vitamin E, it's best to eat fresh food sources. I use 200 iu daily in my diet.

• **Selenium** is a trace mineral that functions in concert with Vitamin E to scavenge free radicals and heavy metals. It is thought to help in the prevention of cancer. It's also important for thyroid function, as it aids in converting T4 to T3. Good sources include Brazil nuts, eggs, lean meats, seafood and legumes. Although the RDA for this mineral is 55mcg, I take 83mcg to insure adequate absorption.

• **Zinc** serves many functions in our body. The bitter metallic taste in your mouth when you eat iodinated table salt is caused by the interaction of zinc in your saliva with the iodine. This metal is important to carbohydrate, fat and protein metabolism and can assist your immune system in fighting a cold. Insulin-like growth factor (IGF-I) is a critical element in bone formation and protein metabolism. Low concentrations of zinc were found to cause low levels of IGF-I in healthy postmenopausal women.[226] In another study, animals switched from preferring carbohydrates to fat after developing a zinc deficiency.[227] Diets high in calcium or calcium containing supplements can reduce the absorption and balance in adults and have a direct effect on hip osteoporosis.[228,222] Foods high in zinc include meat and poultry (especially dark meat), shellfish and legumes. I routinely take 35 mg a day.

• **Vitamin C** has been viewed as the miracle vitamin, curing everything from the common cold to cancer in various doses. Ascorbic acid (Vitamin C) can reduce the risk of gallbladder disease and stones by altering the breakdown of cholesterol.[229-231] Vitamin C levels are associated with a reduction in heart disease and stroke.[232] Postmenopausal women who take at least 500mg of calcium a day with Vitamin C have better collagen formation in bone and tissue.[233] Good sources are fresh fruits, melons, strawberries, broccoli, sweet red and green peppers, tomatoes, brussels sprouts, cabbage and dark leafy greens like chard, kale, collards, spinach, mustard and turnips. The darker or brighter the green pigment, the greater the Vitamin C content. I take 350mg a day.

• **Magnesium** is a mineral which acts to balance the solubility of calcium in urine and tissues. It is vital to metabolism and activates more than 300 different enzymes in the body, particularly those that need the B vitamins for action. It helps to prevent tooth decay by binding calcium to teeth. Good sources are avocados, green vegetables, chocolate (70% cocoa), legumes, nuts and seeds. You should take half as much magnesium as calcium in your supplements, so I use 360mg a day to balance my calcium intake.

• **Vitamin D** is God's gift from sunshine. It regulates phosphorus and calcium metabolism which is important for strong bones. Good sources are cod liver oil, dairy products, butter, eggs, liver, fish such as salmon and of course, sunshine. I only add 33 i.u of cholecalciferol (Vitamin D) to my diet.

• **Biotin** is a highly sulfur containing B vitamin which plays a key role in carbohydrate, fat and protein metabolism. It's what gives rotten eggs their odor! Biotin is important for healthy nails, hair and skin. Good sources are egg yolks, meats, liver, milk, nuts, legumes, peanut butter, chocolate and cauliflower. If you don't eat eggs, consider adding 33 mcg to your diet.

• **Pantothenic acid**, by its Greek name, means "do anything" and that's just about how it works. It's a key component to Coenzyme A which is important to your metabolism of carbohydrates, fats and proteins. Good sources are most fish but all food groups contain some pantothenic acid. I use 166 mg a day.

• **Riboflavin** is nature's way of giving you the

benefits of niacin without the "hot flashes." It's an important B vitamin in the metabolism of tryptophan and has been found to help prevent migraines.[234] Riboflavin is water soluble and works with B6, folate and niacin to maintain the integrity of red blood cells. It also helps to metabolize carbohydrates, fats and proteins. Good sources are liver, eggs, milk, yogurt, cheese, dark green vegetables, spinach and broccoli. I take 66 mg a day.

• **Potassium** is an important mineral in maintaining fluid balance. It also helps our body breakdown carbohydrates and protein. Good sources include fruits, vegetables, dairy products, fish, lean meats and poultry. I take 50mg a day.

• **Chromium** helps to regulate cholesterol and fatty acid production by making the body more sensitive to insulin. It also aids in the digestion of protein. Good sources are unpeeled apples, oysters, nuts, peanut butter, liver and meat. I take 83 mcg in the form of an amino acid chelate.

• **Manganese** is a trace element that appears in a variety of plants and animals. Our bodies use it to activate enzymes that are important in the metabolism of glucose and fatty acids. Good sources are tea, leafy vegetables, nuts, fruits and legumes. I balance my diet with 41 mg.

• **Pyridoxine** or B6 is essential for the metabolism of protein as it helps to convert glycogen into glucose which can be used by your muscles for energy. It is an important co-factor in the regulation of 26 amino-transferases, enzymes that regulate the proper pathways for our neuroendocrine system. If you are deficient in B6, you may form kidney stones when you eat sugars such as fructose or galactose.[235] Women need higher doses of B6 than men because we lose more B6 in our urine.[236] Women taking birth control pills to control excess bleeding can become depleted of B6, which results in disturbances in the metabolism of tryptophan. This can cause depression, anxiety, decreased sex drive and impaired glucose tolerance.[237,238] B6 is important in lowering homocysteine levels in blood. Pyridoxal-5-phosphate, the liver metabolized form of B6, is the active component. However, if you have problems with gastric emptying, you may not be able to absorb B6 from standard vitamins unless it has been treated for absorption in the small intestine or duodenum. I take 20mg enteric coated tablets of Pyridoxal-5-Phosphate twice a day. If you are prone to herpetic outbreaks, don't take B6.

• **Iron deficiency** can alter cholesterol metabolism and predispose you to gallstone formation.[239] If menstruation becomes irregular, monthly blood loss can become severe, creating a deficiency. However, once menstruation stops, higher levels of iron become stored as serum ferritin, which has been shown to be a risk factor for coronary disease.[240] Sources of iron include liver, dried lentils, meat, poultry, broccoli, kale and spinach. Soy products can block the absorption of iron. You should discuss supplementation with your doctor as there are many variables to consider in finding the appropriate dosage for you.

• **Arginine** is an excellent way to handcuff cholesterol and lower your blood pressure. Arginine is an amino acid found in the gelatinous material extracted from bone marrow. It's what gives chicken soup its medicinal properties. The jelly stuff that congeals on your plate contains a growth factor which can slow down the rate of replication of viruses, but more importantly, arginine and vitamin E can block the atherosclerotic plaques that cause blood vessels to go into spasm and deprive your tissue of oxygen.[241] Arginine, especially L-arginine, restores the protective effects of cholecystokinin on the stomach lining.[242] It can also prevent damage to the kidneys by increasing the excretion of nitric oxide metabolites, which can cause scarring of the filtration units called glomeruli.[243] Arginine helps wounds heal from surgery by stimulating the immune system in surgical patients.[244] L-arginine stimulates growth hormone production and inhibits the effect of cortisol on our hormones.[245] A diet rich in carbohydrates has very little arginine, while a protein rich diet has oodles of this amino acid. Soybeans, turkey and chicken contain large amounts of arginine. In fact, soy is exceptionally rich in arginine compared to animal sources. So try taking 500mg of L-arginine twice a day.

As you can see, nutritional support is just another part of "The Goddess Diet" lifestyle. Since everyone can use a helping hand, I designed "Female Formula Stress Tabs" to insure you have all the vitamins and minerals necessary to keep your program on track. Look for information about ordering this supplement in the resource section of this book or online at

http://www.goddessdiet.com

As always, make healthy food your mainstay, but for smart nutrition insurance the right supplements make sense too.

chapter eight

how to chart your own personal journey

Trust me. This next step isn't going to hurt one little bit. All you need is a tape measure to start yourself off on your own personal journey to a slimmer, more vivacious body. So close the door – you don't need any Peeping Toms here and let's get started.

calculating body mass index

Remember that weight is not the factor which determines how healthy you are, but rather three measurements: Body Mass Index, waist circumference and percent body fat. It's easy to measure your waistline – just place the tape around the smallest part of your abdomen above your belly button and below your lowest rib. Go to the chart on the next page and write down your waistline in inches. Now the next two figures are a bit more complicated. To determine your body mass index, you need to take your height and convert it into inches and then meters squared. The chart makes it easier. Now go weigh yourself. Don't worry. I won't look.

I've included detailed instructions in the chart to help you complete your profile. To determine your percent body fat, I highly recommend the new electronic scale by Tanita or the hand held device by Omron. When I used charts, I underestimated my actual body fat by several pounds. Both devices emit a low electrical current that calculates both the percent and actual pounds of fat on your body. Skin calipers can also give you an accurate reading. The gold standard involves submersion in water to determine your precise amount of body fat. Since I am "water soluble" I prefer the electronic scale readings to keep track of my progress.

Now, if you want to know your basal metabolic rate or BMR (how many calories you burn just sitting) multiply your weight in pounds by 11. Add between 400 and 600 calories for mild to intense exercise and routine physical activity and you have a rough idea of how many 250 calorie meals you need in a day just to maintain your weight. Once you are armed with this information, you are ready to proceed to the next step.

body mass index

	21	22	23	24	25	26	27	28	29	30
5'0"	107	112	118	123	128	133	138	143	148	158
5'1"	111	116	122	127	132	137	143	148	153	158
5'2"	115	120	126	131	136	142	147	153	158	164
5'3"	118	124	130	135	141	146	152	158	163	169
5'4"	122	128	134	140	145	151	157	163	169	174
5'5"	126	132	138	144	150	156	162	168	174	180
5'6"	130	136	142	148	155	161	167	173	179	186
5'7"	134	140	146	153	159	166	172	178	185	191
5'8"	138	144	151	158	164	171	177	184	190	197
5'9"	142	149	155	162	169	176	182	189	196	203
5'10"	146	153	160	167	174	181	188	195	202	207
5'11"	150	157	165	172	179	186	193	200	208	215

1. Waist _____ inches
Goal: Under 30 inches

2. Height _____ inches
(multiply feet by 12 and add
the rest as inches)

_____ meters² To convert to meters, multiply
inches by 0.0254 then multiply
that number against itself

*Example 62 inches x 0.0254=1.5748
x 1.5748=2.479 meters²*

3. Weight _____ pounds To convert to
kilograms, divide
by 2.2 _____ kg

4. BMI = kg/m2 _____ Simply take #3
divided by #2
Goal: Under 25 kg/m2

5. Percent body fat _____
Goal: Under 25%

6. BMR = _____ calories
(weight in pounds x 11)

Add 400/600/1000 calories for degree of exercise,
routine physical activity and divide by 250 for the
number of mini meals in a day to maintain your weight.

Calories/250 = _____ mini meals/day

the family tree

I always asked my patients about the risks hiding in their family tree, specifically what illnesses occurred and the cause of any family member's death. More than 3,000 ailments are known to be inherited, including heart disease, cancer, diabetes, arthritis, Alzheimer's, even alcoholism, depression, thyroid disease and schizophrenia. Take time to fill this form out for both sides of your family and make copies for your children. It will make your motivation even stronger for losing weight and staying healthy.

old mother hubbard

I always clean out my cupboards on days when my hormones are really low, usually just before my period. It seems changes in serotonin cause an obsessive cleaning nature in women at this time, so take advantage of the situation and remove temptation, in the form of high glycemic carbohydrates, from your shelves. There is no truth to the rumor that calories are afraid of heights and will leap out of food if stored on the top shelf. Go on...just throw them away.

- Designate a specific cupboard just for your own food items and place any cereals or bread in another cupboard for your family to use.

- Replace cooking oils with olive oil, canola and peanut oil.

- Stock up on spices and teas and get rid of cans of vegetables you've been saving since the beginning of the world.

- Check labels for corn syrup or MSG and eliminate them from your personal cupboard.

Once you've got this situation in hand, let's deal with the shopping list.

your family health history

This blank genogram has room for only your own family history. But you can photo copy the page, add your spouse's family, and combine the two for your children's full health history. Squeeze in extra names, of course, if you have an especially large family. When your genogram is complete, give your doctor a copy for your medical files and make separate copies for your spouse's and children's files. Store another copy for each of your children and update it periodically.

Name of person submitting genogram ————————————

Date ————————————————————————

Address —————————————————————————

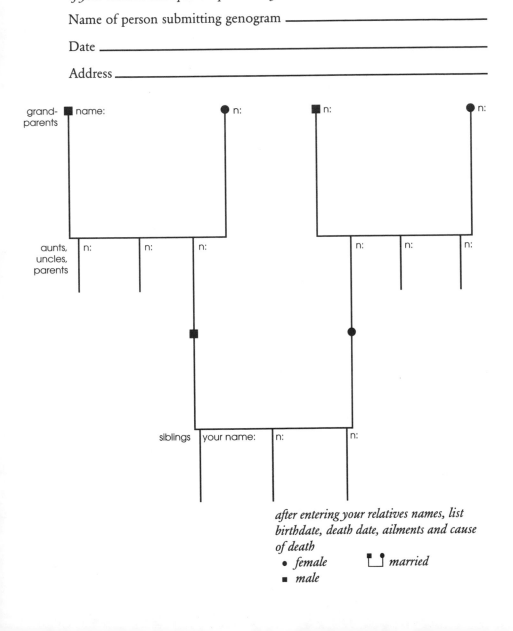

grand-parents ■ name: ● n: ■ n: ● n:

aunts, uncles, parents   n: n: n: n: n: n:

siblings   your name: n: n:

after entering your relatives names, list birthdate, death date, ailments and cause of death
- *female*   ⌐⌐ *married*
- *male*

to market to market

Copy the list of high glycemic carbohydrates on page 46 and keep them with you in the grocery store. It's important in starting The Goddess Diet that you understand which carbohydrates have the ability to raise your blood sugar higher than the Empire State Building if you want to lose weight.

• Choose a wide variety of produce and try to avoid frozen or canned vegetables.

• Compare the grams of carbohydrates that come from sugar in any reduced fat dairy products versus the full fat versions to be certain you're not substituting sugar for fat.

• Lean meats usually come from the loin, so choose filet, pork loin and sirloin instead of ribs and heavily marbled meats.

• Select fish that is fresh, not frozen whenever possible and try to include at least one serving of tuna or salmon each week in your meal plan.

• If you're looking for additional non-fat protein sources, purchase whey and soy protein powders to add to soups, mayonnaise and dressings.

• Corn syrup is contained in an amazing number of soups and drinks, including orange juice concentrate, so be certain to read the labels before putting any new products into your cart.

• Purchase low fructose energy bars and keep one in your purse at all times so you don't accidentally skip a meal. It's saved me from many a munchy madness attack that would have overdrawn my carbohydrate reserve account.

eating out

Portion control is probably the hardest part of eating out, with today's restaurants vying to win the Gordita Grande award when it comes to a main course. The simplest way to overcome this is to order two appetizers and request steamed vegetables as a side dish. Don't forget to eat a salad but demurely pass on the bread. The only time I have dessert is in a restaurant and I treat myself to the most appetizing one on the menu. Remember, the composition of the previous meal affects your next one, so don't be afraid to make an occasional withdrawal on that carbohydrate account.

urge to splurge

You've been great on The Goddess Diet but you're dying for some rice or bread. Can you eat it? Of course. You can do anything you want. But here is how I dealt with the occasional craving. I prepared as much of the food as my eyes told me I wanted, then put the entire serving on my plate along with my protein, fat and low glycemic carbs. I only allowed myself one high glycemic food at a meal every three days. It seemed after a few mouthfuls I didn't need any more to satisfy my urge to splurge. So don't deny yourself any food on the shopping list if you have a craving for it. Just remember – each time you eat a high glycemic carb it's like putting 3 tablespoons of corn syrup in your mouth.

charting your progress

Don't become obsessed about daily weight checks. Fluid levels fluctuate daily in your body and you can lose or gain a pound without having metabolized any fat. I recommend you weigh yourself once a week at the same time of day and take an inventory of your waistline every week. Notice how your clothes fit instead of where the needle on the scale is bouncing. It's a much better indicator of losing fat. Write down your weekly values and compare them after one month. I think you'll be pleased with the results you've achieved by not starving or denying yourself.

a final word

The ability to remain naturally slim, ageless and healthy is within the practical reach of any woman, especially once you understand the unique differences in female metabolism. By using the principles in The Goddess Diet Plan, you can regain the vitality and shape of your youth without the need for pills or surgery. There's no magic involved in becoming a goddess...just a realization that low protein, high carbohydrate, low fat diets are the culprit in making women age faster by increasing the risk of damage to our bodies from uncontrolled blood sugar that can lead to heart disease, strokes and cancer. You have been given the power to control your health through the knowledge I have shared with you in this book. If you use this gift wisely, you will remain naturally slim, healthy and sensuous...at any age!

appendix a
resources for living

the goddess diet website

If you are interested in learning more about the impact of diet on women's hormones, visit my website at

www.goddessdiet.com

where you will find up to date news articles, discussions about the latest scientific research, a newsletter and products of interest to us. You can order personally autographed copies of "The Goddess Diet", motivational audio tapes along with my nutritional supplements "Female Formula Stress Tabs" and "Pyridoxal-5 Phosphate" by calling

1-800-554-3335 in the United States

or

310 471-2375
if you do not have access to the internet.

Share your personal experience with The Goddess Diet Plan on my message board and swap recipes and support with each other. It can be just the helping hand you need!

female formula stress tabs
60 tablets

Two tablets contain:

Beta Carotene	5000 i.u.
D-alpha Tocopherol Acetate	200 i.u.
Sodium Selenite	83 mcg
Zinc Gluconate	35 mg
Vit. C (from ascorbyl palmitate and ascorbic acid)	350 mg
Calcium Carbonate	750 mg
Magnesium Hydroxide	360 mg
Vit. D3 (cholecalciferol)	33 i.u.
Biotin	33 mcg
D-Calcium Pantothenate	166 mg
Riboflavin	66 mg
Potassium Chloride	50 mg
Chromium (amino acid chelate)	83 mcg
Manganese Gluconate	41 mg

pyridoxal-5-phosphate
30 tablets

One tablet contains:

Pyridoxal-5-Phosphate (enteric coated)	20mg

All supplements are 100% natural and free of yeast, corn, sugar, starch, soy, flavors, colors, preservatives, wheat or milk derivatives. All orders are shipped Priority Mail.

body fat monitors

The Tanita Body Fat Monitor/Scale is available at Macy's and other large department stores. The scale measures both weight and body fat in 30 seconds and is programmable for up to four people. It retails for $149.95.

Omron makes a portable hand held body fat analyzer that works on the same principle as the Tanita model. It retails for $129.95 at The Sharper Image and several other electronic stores.

- Call 1-800-634-4350 for a distributor near you.

the goddess diet balancer

The Goddess Diet Balancer works as your personal nutritionist, offering you an easy, quick way to personalize your own weight loss program. This software program counts more than calories; it fully examines your new healthy lifestyle by tracking your age, weight, exercise/activity level and diet goals. Just like a personal nutritionist, The Goddess Diet Balancer helps plan meals, graphs and charts your daily intake, helping you keep track of your diet and progress. You can print an exercise log, progress graphs, average your daily, weekly intake and even print out a customized shopping list.

A personal nutritionist can be costly. With The Goddess Diet Balancer you can benefit for years to come with no additional cost. Whether you are trying to lose weight, follow a special diet or just want to keep track of calories and nutrients consumed, The Goddess Diet Balancer will make it possible to have accurate and complete nutritional data at your fingertips. The program is easy to install and comes with a complete manual as well as free on-line help.

You can obtain The Goddess Diet Balancer CD-ROM in both Windows and Mac formats by calling **1-800-554-3335**

or

by contacting my website
http://www.goddessdiet.com

spices

Purchasing new, exotic spices can lend a real zip to foods while keeping the fat low. One of the best sources is Penzeys Spice catalog. You can order their catalog on line at:

- Penzeys Spices
  www.penzeys.com
  414 679-7207.

For Allepo, pasilla and ancho chili powder, Dean and Deluca is an excellent resource. You can order online at:

- Dean and Deluca
  www.dean-deluca-napavalley.com
  707 967-9880.

Other sources for exotic spices are:
- Kalustyan
  123 Lexington Ave
  New York, NY 10016
  212 685-3451

- Sultan's Delight
  P.O. Box 090302
  Brooklyn, NY 11209
  800 852-6844
  718 745-6844
  Fax 718 745-2563

- The Spice House
  1031 N. Old World Third St
  Milwaukee, WI 53203
  414 272-0977

- Uwajimaya
  800 889-1928

An excellent source for asian spices, such as chinese brown bean paste, star anise, fish sauce, chili paste.

- Foods of India
  212 683-4419

Sadaf brand pomegranate paste for Middle Eastern dishes

- Chile Today—Hot Tamale
  800 468-7377

Dried New Mexican red chilis

- Kitchen Market
  212 243-4433

A great source for banana leaves and dried ancho chilis if you don't have a Latino shop nearby.

- Adriana's Caravan
  409 Vanderbilt St
  Brooklyn, NY 11218
  718 436-8565

This store will ship fresh curry leaves, tamarind concentrate, dried pomegrante seeds and brown mustard seeds.

- Frieda's
  P.O. Box 58488
  Los Angeles, Calif. 90058
  800-241-1771
  http://www.friedas.com

Kaboucha squash, chilis and wax peppers can be found at this unique supplier.

teas

One of my favorite teas is made by Bernardaud's of France. It's a caramel tea and is rich in flavor, even when laced with a little milk. You can order it from:

- La Cucina Rustica
  cyberbaskets.com/cbdocs/items/be9003c.htm
  9950 West Lawrence Avenue, Suite 202
  Schiller Park, IL 60176 USA
  800 796-0116 – Customer Service Department

Stash makes a Mango Passion Fruit tea available in grocery stores and Ceylon Passion has a delightful

Passion Fruit Papaya tea combination. A mixture of black teas with fruit extract, they make delightful iced teas. All are caffeine free and available in your grocery store. Tejava is a delicious micro brewed tea made entirely from the top leaves of each branch picked only from May through October. If you can't find it in your grocery store, call 1-800-4-GEYSER

tomatoes

There is nothing better than fresh tomatoes, but the organic canned tomatoes seasoned with sea salt by Muir Glen do well in a pinch. If you don't find them in your grocery store, call or write

- Muir Glen
  P.O. Box 1498
  Sacramento, California
  707 778-7801
  www.muirglen.com *has a store locator on the site*

sea salt

Searching for specialty sea salts has become a hobby of mine and I will share with you my secret sources.

- The Baker's Catalogue
  P.O. Box 876
  Norwich, VT 05055-0876
  800 827-6836
  http://www.kingarthurflour.com

This company sells Maldon Crystal sea salt, Celtic Grey and Fleur de sel de Guaerande, the most expensive type of salt, harvested under special conditions.

- Zingerman's
  422 Detroit St.
  Ann Arbor, MI 48104
  888 636-8162

This is another source for Fleur de sel de Guerande.

- Corti Brothers
5810 Folsom Blvd.
Sacramento, Calif 95822
800 509-FOOD

This company carries Sicilian sea salt and Japanese Oshima Island salt.

the greatest grater

Microplane has found a new use for a woodworker's rasp – zesting citrus, cheese and chocolate. These blades come in fine or coarse ratings which can be simply changed out as needed. You can purchase them from Sur La Table or from Microplane for under $15.

- Microplane
Lee Valley Tools
800 871-8158
http://www.microplane.com

japanese mandoline

This nifty little device is like an apple corer only standing upright. It can make oodles of noodles out of any hard vegetable with just a turn of the handle. You can purchase one from Sur La Table.

- Sur La Table
800 221-5786

chocolate soap

I'm all in a lather over this find! Fleurs de Chocolat has bath products composed of cocoa extract, pear and orange essences that could send Casanova into a swoon. I adore their Chocolate soap.

- Fleur de Chocolat
800 373-7420

recumbent bikes

To find a distributor for the BikeE CT 2.0, call:

- BikeE
  1-800-231-3136
  5125 S W Hout
  Corvallis, Oregon 97333
It retails for $650.

pilates®

If you're looking for books, videos and equipment in order to perform Pilates® contact:

- Current Concepts
  1-800-240-3539

They have several books available. Be sure and ask for this one:

- Body Control Pilates
  by Lynne Robinson and
  Gordon Thomson
  BainBridge Books, 1998

Here are other resources for this exercise program:

- PhysicalMind Institute
  1-800-505-1990

- Pilates Studio
  1-800-474-5283
  www.pilates-studio.com
They sell a foldable home exercise reformer for stretching

To get started on exercising, just go to any bookstore and stand in front of the health and fitness section. You will be amazed at how many ways you can tone and firm your body.

I recommend the following books for their clean, simple approach to understanding weight training and body shaping.

- Body Shaping
  by Michael Yessis, PhD.,
  Rodale Press, 1994

- Callanetics
  by Callan Pinckney,
  Perigee Books, 1997

- Power Yoga
  by Beryl Bender Birch,
  Fireside, 1995

- A Woman's Book of Strength
  by Karen Andes,
  Perigee Books, 1995

- Strong Women Stay Young
  by Miriam Nelson
  Bantam Books, 1997

If you are interested in reading about the health benefits of arginine, pick up this book:

- The Arginine Solution
  by Robert Fried Ph.D.
  and Woodson Merrell, MD.,
  Warner Books, 1999

There is only one book every person who has ever suffered from kidney stones should have in their home health library. It's even recommended by Former Surgeon General C. Everett Koop:

- The Kidney Stones Handbook,
  Gail Savitz and Stephen Leslie, M.D.,
  Four Geez Press, 1999
  1-800-2kidney
  916 781-3440

1911 Douglass Blvd #85
Roseville, Ca 95661
ggolomb@ns.net

If you want to see the full listing of foods tested to date and their GI ratings, read this book:

- The Glucose Revolution:
  The Authoritative Guide to the Glycemic Index
  by Jennie Brand Miller, Thomas Wolever and
  and Kaye Foster-Powell
  Marlowe & Co., 1999

If you want to try Prayer-walking, read this book:

- The Complete Guide to Prayer-Walking
  by Linus Mundy
  Crossroads Publications, 1997

These books on breathing will give you a practical guide to deep relaxation and much more:

- The Breathing Book
  by Donna Farhi,
  Owl Books, 1996

- The Tao of Natural Breathing
  by Dennis Lewis,
  Mountain Wind Publishing, 1997

- Conscious Breathing
  by Gay Hendricks, Ph.D.,
  Bantam Books, 1995

appendix b

references

1. Kuczmarski, R., *et al., Increasing prevalence of overweight among US adults: the National Health and Nutrition Examination Surveys, 1960-1991.* JAMA, 1994. 272: p. 205-211.

2. LaCroix, A. *and et al., Healthy Aging: A Woman's Issue.* West. J. Med., 1997. 167(Oct): p. 220-232.

3. Tarnopolsky, M.A., *et al., Carbohydrate loading and metabolism during exercise in men and women.* J Appl Physiol, 1995. 78(4): p. 1360-8.

4. Geary, N., *Estradiol and the control of eating.* Appetite, 1997. 29(3): p. 386.

5. Ganesan, R., *The aversive and hypophagic effects of estradiol.* Physiol Behav, 1994. 55(2): p. 279-85.

6. Petroianu, A., *Gallbladder emptying in perimenopausal women.* Med Hypotheses, 1989. 30(2): p. 129-30.

7. Lam, W.F., *et al., Influence of hyperglycemia on the satiating effect of CCK in humans.* Physiol Behav, 1998. 65(3): p. 505-11.

8. Ortega, R.M., *et al., Differences in diet and food habits between patients with gallstones and controls.* J Am Coll Nutr, 1997. 16(1): p. 88-95.

9. Attili, A.F., *et al., Diet and gallstones in Italy: the cross-sectional MICOL results.* Hepatology, 1998. 27(6):p.1492-8.

10. Caroli-Bosc, F.X., *et al., Cholelithiasis and dietary risk factors: an epidemiologic investigation in Vidauban, Southeast France.* General Practitioner's Group of Vidauban. Dig Dis Sci, 1998. 43(9): p. 2131-7.

11. Gazizova, R.R., A.V. Novikova, and M.A. Vinogradova, *Age-related features of inflammatory and immune responses of the gastric mucosa in women with chronic gastritis.* Patol Fiziol Eksp Ter, 1995(4): p. 32-4.

12. Konturek, J.W., *et al., Physiological role of cholecystokinin in gastroprotection in humans.* Am J Gastroenterol, 1998. 93(12): p. 2385-90.

13. Nilsson, P., *et al., Social and biological predictors of early menopause: a model for premature aging.* J Intern Med, 1997. 242(4): p. 299-305.

14. Wilson, J. and D. Foster, *Williams Textbook of Endocrinology.* 8 ed. 1992, Philadelphia: W.B. Saunders.

15. Rosano, G., *et al., Syndrome X in women is associated with estrogen*

deficiency. Eur Heart J, 1995. 16(5): p. 610-14.

16. Spencer, C.P., I.F. Godsland, and J.C. Stevenson, *Is there a menopausal metabolic syndrome?* Gynecol Endocrinol, 1997. 11(5): p. 341-55.

17. Colombel, A. and B. Charbonnel, *Weight gain and cardiovascular risk factors in the postmenopausal women.* Hum Reprod, 1997. 12 Suppl 1: p. 134-45.

18. Gensini, G.F., M. Comeglio, and A. Colella, *Classical risk factors and emerging elements in the risk profile for coronary artery disease.* Eur Heart J, 1998. 19 Suppl A: p. A53-61.

19. Goodman, M.T., et al., *The association of diet, obesity, and breast cancer in Hawaii.* Cancer Epidemiol Biomarkers Prev, 1992. 1(4): p. 269-75.

20. Legato, M.J., *Cardiovascular disease in women: gender-specific aspects of hypertension and the consequences of treatment.* J Womens Health, 1998. 7(2): p. 199-209.

21. Maurer, K.R., *et al., Risk factors for gallstone disease in the Hispanic populations of the United States.* Am J Epidemiol, 1990. 131(5): p. 836-44.

22. Large, V. and P. Arner, *Regulation of lypolysis in humans. Pathophysiological modulation in obesity, diabetes and hyperlipidaemia.* Diabetes Metab, 1998. 24(5): p. 409-18.

23. Anate, M., A. Olatinwo, and A. Omesina, *Obesity—an overview.* West Afr J Med, 1998. 17(4): p. 248-54.

24. Carey, D.G., *et al., Abdominal fat and insulin resistance in normal and overweight women: Direct measurements reveal a strong relationship in subjects at both low and high risk of NIDDM.* Diabetes, 1996. 45(5): p. 633-8.

25. Goldsmith, H., *The Omentum.* 1990, New York: Springer-Verlag.

26. Bjorntorp, P., *The regulation of adipose tissue distribution in humans.* Int J Obes Relat Metab Disord, 1996. 20(4): p. 291-302.

27. Bronnegard, M., P. Arner, and L. Hellstrom, *et al., Glucocorticoid receptor messenger ribonucleic acid in different regiosn of human adipose tissue.* Endocrinol, 1990. 127: p. 1689-1696.

28. Iannoli, P., *et al., Glucocorticoids upregulate intestinal nutrient transport in a time-dependent and substrate-specific fashion.* Gastrointest Surg, 1998. 2(5): p. 449-57.

29. Bongain, A., V. Isnard, and J.Y. Gillet, *Obesity in obstetrics and gynaecology.* Eur J Obstet Gynecol Reprod Biol, 1998. 77(2): p. 217-28.

30. Samojlik, E., M. Kirschner, and D. Silber, *et al., Elevated production and metabolic clearance rates of androgens in morbidly obese women.* J Clin Endocrinol Metab, 1984. 59: p. 949.

31. Kirschner, M. and J. Jacobs, *Combined ovarian and adrenal vein catheterization to determine the site of androgen overproduction in hirsute women.* J Clin Endocrino Metab, 1971. 1(33): p. 199.

32. Barbieri, R., *Adipose Tissue and Reproduction.* Prog Reprod Biol Med, ed. R. Frisch. Vol. 14. 1990, Basel: Karger. 42-57.

33. Lemieux, S., et al., *A single threshold value of waist girth identifies normal-weight and overweight subjects with excess visceral adipose tissue.* Am J CLin Nutr, 1996. 64: p. 685-93.

34. Lyu, L.C., et al., *Relationship of body fat distribution with cardiovascular risk factors in healthy Chinese.* Ann Epidemiol, 1994. 4(6): p. 434-44.

35. Panotopoulos, G., et al., *Weight gain at the time of menopause.* Hum Reprod, 1997. 12 Suppl 1: p. 126-33.

36. Stevenson, J.C., et al., *HRT mechanisms of action: carbohydrates.* Int J Fertil Menopausal Stud, 1994. 39(Suppl 1): p. 50-5.

37. Gaspard, U.J., J.M. Gottal, and F.A. van den Brule, *Postmenopausal changes of lipid and glucose metabolism: a review of their main aspects.* Maturitas, 1995. 21(3):p. 71-8.

38. Wild, R., P. Painter, and P. Coulson, et al., *Lipoprotein lipid concentrations and cardiovascular risk in women with polycystic ovarian syndrome.* J Clin Endocrinol Metab, 1985. 61: p. 946.

39. Rexrode, K., et al., *Abdominal adiposity and coronary heart diease in women.* JAMA, 1998. 280: p. 1843-1848.

40. Williams, M.J., et al., *Regional fat distribution in women and risk of cardiovascular disease.* Am J Clin Nutr, 1997. 65(3): p. 855-60.

41. Harris, M., *Epidemiological correlates of NIDDM in Hispanics, whites and blacks in the US population.* Diabetes Care, 1991. 14 (Suppl 3): p. S639-S648.

42. Gavin, J., *The role of the gastrointestinal tract and alpha-glucosidase inhibition in Type II diabetes.* Drug Benefits Trends, 1996(Supp 8E): p. 18-26.

43. Jarrett, R., H. Keen, and J. Fulley, et. al., *Worsening to diabetes in men with impaired glucose tolerance (borderline diabetes).* Diabetologia, 1979. 16: p. 25-30.

44. Redberg, R.F., *Coronary artery disease in women: understanding the diagnostic and management pitfalls.* Medscape Womens Health, 1998. 3(5): p. 1.

45. Wenger, N.K., *The High Risk of CHD for Women: Understanding Why Prevention Is Crucial.* Medscape Womens Health, 1996. 1(11):p. 6.

46. Kahn, H.S., L.M. Tatham, and C.W. Heath, Jr., *Contrasting factors associated with abdominal and peripheral weight gain among adult women.* Int J Obes Relat Metab Disord, 1997. 21(10): p. 903-11.

47. Bresnick, J. and T. Hanlon, *Custom tailored hormone therapy*, in Prevention. 1995. p. 65-73.

48. Knight., L., et al., *Delayed gastric emptying and decreased antral contractility in normal premenopausal women compared with men.* Am J Gastroenterol, 1997. 92(6): p. 968-75.

49. Weber, E. and H.J. Ehrlein, *Relationships between gastric emptying and intestinal absorption of nutrients and energy in mini pigs.* Dig Dis Sci, 1998. 43(6): p. 1141-53.

50. Raskin, P., *et al.*, *Abnormal alpha cell function in human diabetes: the response to oral protein.* Am J Med, 1978. 64(6): p. 988-97.

51. Wagner, R. and J. Warkany, *Untersuchungen uber den zuckerbildenden Wert der Gemuse in der Diabetikerkost.* Z Kinderheilk, 1927. 44: p. 322.

52. Crapo, P., G. Reaven, and J. Olefsky, *Plasma glucose and insulin responses to orally administered simple and complex carbohydrates.* Diabetes, 1976. 25: p. 741-747.

53. Wolever, T.M., *et al.*, *Glycemic index of foods in individual subjects.* Diabetes Care, 1990. 13(2): p. 126-32.

54. Jenkins, D., T. Wolever, and R. Taylor, *Glycemic index of foods: a physiological basis for carbohydrate exchange.* Am J Clin Nutr, 1981. 34: p. 362-6.

55. Juliano, B.O., *et al.*, *Properties of Thai cooked rice and noodles differing in glycemic index in noninsulin-dependent diabetics [published erratum appears in Plant Foods Hum Nutr 1990 Jul;40(3):231-2].* Plant Foods Hum Nutr, 1989. 39(4): p. 369-74.

56. Wolever, T., *et al.*, *Glycaemic index of 102 complex carbohydrate foods in patients with diabetes.* Nutr Res, 1994. 14: p. 651-669.

57. Gannon, M. and F. Nuttall, *Factors affecting interpretation of postprandial glucose and insulin areas.* Diabetes Care, 1987. 10: p. 759-763.

58. Melanson, K., *et al.*, *Blood glucose and hormonal response to small and large meals in healthy young and old women.* J Gerontol: Biol Sc, 1998. 53A: p. 4.

59. Wolever, T.M., *The glycemic index.* World Rev Nutr Diet, 1990. 62: p. 120-85.

60. Nuttall, F., *et al.*, *Effect of protein ingestion on the glucose and insulin response to a standardized oral glucose load.* Diabetes Care, 1984. 7: p. 465-470.

61. Smith, G.P. and J. Gibbs, *Are gut peptides a new class of anorectic agents?* Am J Clin Nutr, 1992. 55(1 Suppl): p. 283S-285S.

62. Welch, I., *et al.*, *Duodenal and ileal lipid suppresses postprandial blood glucose an dinsulin responses in man: possible implications for the dietary managment of diabetes mellitus.* Clin Sci, 1987. 72: p. 209-216.

63. Collier, G., T. Wolever, and D. Jenkins, *Concurrent ingestion of fat and reduction in starch content impairs carbohydrate tolerance to subsequent meals.* Am J Clin Nutr, 1987. 45: p. 963-969.

64. Wolever, T.M. and C. Bolognesi, *Prediction of glucose and insulin responses of normal subjects after consuming mixed meals varying in energy, protein, fat, carbohydrate and glycemic index.* J Nutr, 1996. 126(11): p. 2807-12.

65. Jenkins, D., *et al.*, *Metabolic effects of a low-glycemic-index diet.* Am J Clin Nutr, 1987. 46(6): p. 968-75.

66. Jenkins, D., T. Wolever, and G. Buckley, *et al.*, *Low glycemic index starchy foods in the diabetic diet.* AM J Clin Nutr, 1988. 48: p. 248-254.

67. Jenkins, D., *et al.*, *Nibbling versus gorging: metabolic advantages of increased meal frequency.* N Engl J Med, 1989. 321(14): p. 929-34.

68. Jenkins, D.J., *et al.*, *Low glycemic index: lente carbohydrates and physiological effects of altered food frequency.* Am J Clin Nutr, 1994. 59(3 Suppl): p. 706S-709S.

69. Leibowitz, S.F., A. Akabayashi, and J. Wang, *Obesity on a high-fat diet: role of hypothalamic galanin in neurons of the anterior paraventricular nucleus projecting to the median eminence.* J Neurosci, 1998. 18(7): p. 2709-19.

70. Jenkins, D., *et al.*, *"Nibbling versus gorging": metabolic advantages of increased meal frequency.* N Eng J Med, 1989. 321: p. 929-34.

71. Himaya, A. and J. Louis-Sylvestre, *The effect of soup on satiation.* Appetite, 1998. 30(2): p. 199-210.

72. Wolever, T.M., *et al.*, *Second-meal effect: low-glycemic-index foods eaten at dinner improve subsequent breakfast glycemic response.* Am J Clin Nutr, 1988. 48(4): p. 1041-7.

73. Parodi, P.W., *The French paradox unmasked: the role of folate.* Med Hypotheses, 1997. 49(4): p. 313-8.

74. Drewnowski, A., *et al.*, *Diet quality and dietary diversity in France: implications for the French paradox.* J Am Diet Assoc, 1996. 96(7): p. 663-9.

75. Hercberg, S., *et al.*, *Vitamin status of a healthy French population: dietary intakes and biochemical markers.* Int J Vitam Nutr Res, 1994. 64(3): p. 220-32.

76. Monneuse, M.O., F. Bellisle, and G. Koppert, *Eating habits, food and health related attitudes and beliefs reported by French students.* Eur J Clin Nutr, 1997. 51(1): p. 46-53.

77. Chatenoud, L., *et al.*, *Whole grain food intake and cancer risk.* Int J Cancer, 1998. 77(1): p. 24-8.

78. La Vecchia, C. and A. Tavani, *Fruit and vegetables, and human cancer.* Eur J Cancer Prev, 1998. 7(1): p. 3-8.

79. Michaud, C., *et al.*, *Food habits, consumption, and knowledge of a low-income French population.* Sante Publique, 1998. 10(3): p. 333-47.

80. Jeffery, R.W. and S.A. French, *Epidemic obesity in the United States: are fast foods and television viewing contributing?* Am J Public Health, 1998. 88(2): p. 277-80.

81. Larson, D.E., *et al.*, *Dietary fat in relation to body fat and intra-abdominal adipose tissue: a cross-sectional analysis.* Am J Clin Nutr, 1996. 64(5): p. 677-84.

82. Ginsberg, H.N., *et al.*, *Effects of reducing dietary saturated fatty acidson plasma lipids and lipoproteins in healthy subjects: the DELTA Study, protocol 1.* Arterioscler Thromb Vasc Biol, 1998. 18(3): p. 441-9.

83. O'Bryne, D.J., S.F. O'Keefe, and R.B. Shireman, *Low-fat, monounsaturate-rich diets reduce susceptibility of low density lipoproteins to peroxidation ex vivo.* Lipids, 1998. 33(2): p. 149-57.

84. Low, C., E. Grossman, and B. Gumbiner, *Potentiation of effects of weight loss by monunsaturated fatty acids in obese NIDDM patients.* Diabetes, 1996. 45: p. 569-575.

85. O'Byrne, D.J., D.A. Knauft, and R.B. Shireman, *Low fat-monounsaturated rich diets containing higholeic peanuts improve serum lipoprotein profiles.* Lipids, 1997. 32(7): p. 687-95.

86. Trautwein, E.A., *et al., Effect of dietary fats rich in lauric, myristic, palmitic, oleic or linoleic acid on plasma, hepatic and biliary lipids in cholesterol-fed hamsters.* Br J Nutr, 1997. 77(4): p. 605-20.

87. Association, A.M., American Medical Association Essential Guide to Menopause. 1 ed. 1998, New York: Pocket Books. 253.

88. Jeppesen, J., *et al., Effects of low-fat, high-carbohydrate diets on risk factors for ischemic heart disease in postmenopausal women [published erratum appears in Am J Clin Nutr 1997 Aug;66(2):437].* Am J Clin Nutr, 1997. 65(4): p. 1027-33.

89. Grundy, S., *Comparison of monounsaturated fatty acids and carbohydrates for lowering plasma cholesterol.* N Eng J Med, 1986. 314: p. 745-748.

90. Garg, A., *et al., Comparison of a high-carbohydrate diet with a high-monounsaturated-fat diet in patients with non-insulin-dependent diabetes mellitus.* N Engl J Med, 1988. 319(13): p. 829-34.

91. Bush, T., E. Barrett-Connor, and L *et. al. Cowan, Cardiovascular mortality and noncontraceptive use of estogen in women: results from the Lipid Research Clinics Program Follow-up Study.* Circulation, 1987. 75: p. 1102-9.

92. Brunner, D., J. Weisbort, and N. Meshulam, *et al., Meshulam, Relation of serum total cholesterol and high-density lipoprotein cholesterol percentage to the incidence of definite coronary events:twenty-year follow-up of the Donolo-Tel Aviv prospetive coronary artery disease study.* Am J Cardiol, 1987. 59: p. 1271-6.

93. Bass, K *et al., Plasma lipoprotein levels as predictors of cardio-vascular death in women.* Arch Intern Med, 1993. 153: p. 2209-16.

94. Stensvold, I., *et al., Non-fasting serum triglyceride concentration and mortality from coronary heart disease and any cause in middle-aged Norwegian women.* Br J Med, 1993. 307: p. 1318-22.

95. Sugano, M., *Characteristics of fats in Japanese diets and current recommendations.* Lipids, 1996. 31 Suppl: p.S283-6.

96. Weisburger, J.H., *Dietary fat and risk of chronic disease: mechanistic insights from experimental studies.* J Am Diet Assoc, 1997. 97(7 Suppl): p. S16-23.

97. Masai, M., H. Ito, and T. Kotake, *Effect of dietary intake on urinary oxalate excretion in calcium renal stone formers.* Br J Urol, 1995. 76(6): p. 692-6.

98. Schwille, P., E. Hanisch, and D. Scholz, *Postprandial hyperoxaluria and intestinal oxalate absorption in idiopathic renal stone disease.* J Urol, 1984. 132: p. 650-5.

99. Trinchierti, A., *et al.*, *The influence of diet on urinary risk factors for stones in healthy subjects and idiopathic renal calcium stone formers.* Br J Urol, 1991. 67: p. 230-6.

100. Curhan, G.C., *et al.*, *Comparison of dietary calcium with supplemental calcium and other nutrients as factors affecting the risk for kidney stones in women.* Ann Intern Med, 1997. 126(7): p. 497-504.

101. Curhan, G.C., *et al.*, *Beverage use and risk for kidney stones in women.* Ann Intern Med, 1998. 128(7): p. 534-40.

102. Schubert, W., *et al.*, *Inhibition of 17 beta-estradiol metabolism by grapefruit juice in ovariectomized women.* Maturitas, 1994. 20(2-3): p. 155-63.

103. Pomerleau, J., *et al.*, *Effect of protein intake on glycaemic control and renal function in type 2 (non-insulin-dependent) diabetes mellitus.* Diabetologia, 1993. 36(9): p. 829-34.

104. Preuss, H.G., *et al.*, *Effects of diets high in refined carbohydrates on renal ammonium excretion in rats.* Am J Physiol, 1986. 250(2 Pt 1): p. E156-63

105. Reyes, A.A. and S. Klahr, *Dietary supplementation of L-arginine ameliorates renal hypertrophy in rats fed a high-protein diet.* Proc Soc Exp Biol Med, 1994. 206(2): p.157-61.

106. Lustig, R., R. Hershcopf, and H. Bradlow, *The effects of body weight and diet on estrogen metabolism and estrogen-dependent disease, in Adipose Tissue and Reproduction,* R. Frisch, Editor. 1990, Karger: Basel. p. 107-124.

107. Michnovicz, J., *Environmental modulation of oestrogen metabolism in humans.* Int Clin Nutr Rev, 1987. 7: p. 169-173.

108. Bucala, R., *et al.*, *Increased levels of 16 alpha-hydroxyestrone-modified proteins in pregnancy and in systemic lupus erythematosus.* J Clin Endocrinol Metab, 1985. 60(5): p. 841-7.

109. Fishman, J., J. Schneider, and R. Hershcopf, *et al.*, *Increased estrogen 16 alpha-hydroxylase activity in women with breast and endometrial cancer.* J Steroid Biochem, 1984. 20: p. 1077-1081.

110. Anderson, K.E., *et al.*, *The influence of dietary protein and carbohydrate on the principal oxidative biotransformations of estradiol in normal subjects.* J Clin Endocrinol Metab, 1984. 59(1): p. 103-7.

111. Longcope, C., *et al.*, *The effect of a low fat diet on estrogen metabolism.* J Clin Endocrinol Metab, 1987. 64(6): p. 1246-50.

112. Bradlow, H., R. Hershcopf, and J. Fishman, *Oestradiol 16 alpha-hydroxylase: a risk marker for breast cancer.* Cancer surv, 1986. 5: p. 573-583.

113. Hu, F.B., *et al.*, *Dietary protein and risk of ischemic heart disease in women.* Am J Clin Nutr, 1999. 70(2): p. 221-7.

114. Frost, G., *et al.*, *Glycaemic index as a determinant of serum HDL-cholesterol concentration.* Lancet, 1999. 353(9158): p. 1045-8.

115. Munger, R.G., J.R. Cerhan, and B.C. Chiu, *Prospective study of dietary protein intake and risk of hip fracture in postmenopausal women.* Am J Clin Nutr, 1999. 69(1): p. 147-52.

116. Barzel, U.S. and L.K. Massey, *Excess dietary protein can adversely affect bone.* J Nutr, 1998. 128(6): p. 1051-3.

117. Knight, D.C. and J.A. Eden, *A review of the clinical effects of phytoestrogens.* Obstet Gynecol, 1996. 87(5 Pt 2): p. 897-904.

118. Arjmandi, B.H., et al., *Role of soy protein with normal or reduced isoflavone content in reversing bone loss induced by ovarian hormone deficiency in rats.* Am J Clin Nutr, 1998. 68(6 Suppl): p. 1358S-1363S.

119. Challier, B., J.M. Perarnau, and J.F. Viel, *Garlic, onion and cereal fibre as protective factors for breast cancer: a French case-control study.* Eur J Epidemiol, 1998. 14(8): p. 737-47.

120. Nestel, P.J., et al., *Soy isoflavones improve systemic arterial compliance but not plasma lipids in menopausal and perimenopausal women.* Arterioscler Thromb Vasc Biol, 1997. 17(12): p. 3392-8.

121. Simon, A.H., et al., *Renal haemodynamic responses to a chicken or beef meal in normal individuals.* Nephrol Dial Transplant, 1998. 13(9): p. 2261-4.

122. Anderson, J.W., et al., *Effects of soy protein on renal function and proteinuria in patients with type 2 diabetes.* Am J Clin Nutr, 1998. 68(6 Suppl): p. 1347S-1353S.

123. Murkies, A., *Phytoestrogens—what is the current knowledge?* Aust. Fam Physician, 1998. 27(suppl 1): p. 547-551.

124. Ferraroni, M., et al., *Alcohol consumption and risk of breast cancer: a multicentre Italian case-control study.* Eur J Cancer, 1998. 34(9): p. 1403-9.

125. Oneta, C., et al., *First pass metabolism of ethanol is strikingly influenced by the speed of gastric emptying.* Gut, 1998. 43(5): p. 612-9.

126. Ginsburg, E.S., et al., *The effect of acute ethanol ingestion on estrogen levels in postmenopausal women using transdermal estradiol.* J Soc Gynecol Investig, 1995. 2(1): p. 26-9.

127. Purohit, V., *Moderate alcohol consumption and estrogen levels in post-menopausal women: a review.* Alcohol Clin Exp Res, 1998. 22(5): p. 994-7.

128. Bradley, K.A., et al., *Medical risks for women who drink alcohol.* J Gen Intern Med, 1998. 13(9): p. 627-39.

129. Muti, P., et al., *Alcohol consumption and total estradiol in premenopausal women.* Cancer Epidemiol Biomarkers Prev, 1998. 7(3): p. 189-93.

130. Dallongeville, J., et al., *Influence of alcohol consumption and various beverages on waist girth and waist-to-hip ratio in a sample of French men and women.* Int J Obes Relat Metab Disord, 1998. 22(12): p. 1178-83.

131. Criqui, M.H., *Do known cardiovascular risk factors mediate the effect of alcohol on cardiovascular disease?.* Novartis Found Symp, 1998. 216: p. 159-67.

132. Godfroid, I.O., *Eulogy of wine?.* Presse Med, 1997. 26(40): p. 1971-4.

133. Lloyd, T., et al., *Dietary caffeine intake and bone status of postmeno-pausal women.* Am J Clin Nutr, 1997. 65(6): p. 1826-30.

134. Tavani, A., E. Negri, and C. La Vecchia, *Coffee intake and risk of hip fracture in women in northern Italy.* Prev Med, 1995. 24(4): p. 396-400.

135. Tavani, A., *et al., Coffee consumption and the risk of breast cancer.* Eur J Cancer Prev, 1998. 7(1): p. 77-82.

136. Tavani, A., *et al., Coffee and tea intake and risk of cancers of the colon and rectum: a study of 3,530 cases and 7,057 controls.* Int J Cancer, 1997. 73(2): p. 193-7.

137. Pizziol, A., *et al., Effects of caffeine on glucose tolerance: a placebo-controlled study.* Eur J Clin Nutr, 1998. 52(11): p. 846-9.

138. Kleiner, S.M., *Water: an essential but overlooked nutrient.* J Am Diet Assoc, 1999. 99(2): p. 200-6.

139. Svetkey, L.P., *et al., Preliminary evidence of linkage of salt sensitivity in black Americans at the beta 2-adrenergic receptor locus.* Hypertension, 1997. 29(4): p. 918-22.

140. Chan, T.Y., *et al., Urinary dopamine outputs do not rise in healthy Chinese subjects during gradually increasing oral sodium intake over 8 days.* J Auton Pharmacol, 1996. 16(3): p. 155-9.

141. Iwaoka, T., *et al., The effect of low and high NaCl diets on oral glucose tolerance.* Klin Wochenschr, 1988. 66(16): p. 724-8.

142. Gonzalez Vilchez, F., *et al., Cardiac manifestations of primary hypothyroidism. Determinant factors and treatment response.* Rev Esp Cardiol, 1998. 51(11): p. 893-900.

143. Massoudi, M.S., *et al., Prevalence of thyroid antibodies among healthy middle-aged women. Findings from the thyroid study in healthy women.* Ann Epidemiol, 1995. 5(3): p. 229-33.

144. Nunez, S. and J. Leclere, *Diagnosis of hypothyroidism in the adult.* Rev Prat, 1998. 48(18): p. 1993-8.

145. Stockigt, J.R., *Thyroid disease.* Med J Aust, 1993. 158(11): p. 770-4.

146. Reinhardt, W., *et al., Effect of small doses of iodine on thyroid function in patients with Hashimoto's thyroiditis residing in an area of mild iodine deficiency.* Eur J Endocrinol, 1998. 139(1): p. 23-8.

147. Konno, N., *et al., Association between dietary iodine intake and prevalence of subclinical hypothyroidism in the coastal regions of Japan.* J Clin Endocrinol Metab, 1994. 78(2): p. 393-7.

148. Levi, B. and M.J. Werman, *Long-term fructose consumption accelerates glycation and several age-related variables in male rats.* J Nutr, 1998. 128(9): p. 1442-9.

149. Gannon, M.C., *et al., Stimulation of insulin secretion by fructose ingested with protein in people with untreated type 2 diabetes.* Diabetes Care, 1998. 21(1): p. 16-22.

150. Okuno, G., *et al., Glucose tolerance, blood lipid, insulin and glucagon concentration after single or continuous administration of aspartame in diabetics.* Diabetes Res Clin Pract, 1986. 2(1): p. 23-7.

151. Malaisse, W.J., *et al.*, *Effects of artificial sweeteners on insulin release and cationic fluxes in rat pancreatic islets.* Cell Signal, 1998. 10(10): p. 727-33.

152. Vezina, W.C., *et al.*, *Similarity in gallstone formation from 900 kcal/day diets containing 16 g vs 30 g of daily fat: evidence that fat restriction is not the main culprit of cholelithiasis during rapid weight reduction.* Dig Dis Sci, 1998. 43(3): p. 554-61.

153. Guerguen, L., *Interactions lipides-calcium alimentaires et biodisponibilite du calcium du fromage.* Cah. Nutr. Diet., 1992. XXVII(5): p. 311-314.

154. Teegarden, D., *et al.*, *Previous milk consumption is associated with greater bone density in young women.* Am J Clin Nutr, 1999. 69(5): p. 1014-7.

155. Edes, T.E. and J.H. Shah, *Glycemic index and insulin response to a liquid nutritional formula compared with a standard meal.* J Am Coll Nutr, 1998. 17(1): p. 30-5.

156. Sharma, R.D., T.C. Raghuram, and N.S. Rao, *Effect of fenugreek seeds on blood glucose and serum lipids in type I diabetes.* Eur J Clin Nutr, 1990. 44(4): p. 301-6.

157. Geleijnse, J.M., *et al.*, *Tea flavonoids may protect against atherosclerosis: the Rotterdam Study.* Arch Intern Med, 1999. 159(18): p. 2170-4.

158. Preuss, H.G., *et al.*, *Effects of diets high in refined carbohydrates on renal ammonium excretion in rats.* Am J Physiol, 1986. 250(2 Pt 1): p. E156-63.

159. Wolever, T.M. and J.B. Miller, *Sugars and blood glucose control.* Am J Clin Nutr, 1995. 62(1 Suppl): p. 212S-221S; discussion 221S-227S.

160. Chen, Y.D., *et al.*, *Why do low-fat high-carbohydrate diets accentuate postprandial lipemia in patients with NIDDM?* Diabetes Care, 1995. 18(1): p. 10-6.

161. Ginsberg, H.N., *et al.*, *Increases in dietary cholesterol are associated with modest increases in both LDL and HDL cholesterol in healthy young women.* Arterioscler Thromb Vasc Biol, 1995. 15(2): p. 169-78.

162. Jiang, Y.H., R.B. McGeachin, and C.A. Bailey, *alpha-tocopherol, beta-carotene, and retinol enrichment of chicken eggs.* Poult Sci, 1994. 73(7): p. 1137-43.

163. Kris-Etherton, P.M., *et al.*, *The role of fatty acid saturation on plasma lipids, lipoproteins, and apolipoproteins: I. Effects of whole food diets high in cocoa butter, olive oil, soybean oil, dairy butter, and milk chocolate on the plasma lipids of young men.* Metabolism, 1993. 42(1): p. 121-9.

164. Miller, J. and T. Leeds, *The G.I. Factor: The Glycaemic Index Solution.* 1996: Hodder Healine Asutralia Pty. Ltd.

165. Lewis, S.J., *et al.*, *Lower serum oestrogen concentrations associated with faster intestinal transit.* Br J Cancer, 1997. 76(3): p. 395-400.

166. McGinnis, J.M., *The public health burden of a sedentary lifestyle.* Med Sci Sports Exerc, 1992. 24(6 Suppl): p. S196-200.

167. McTiernan, A., *et al.*, *Prevalence and correlates of recreational physical activity in women aged 50-64 years.* Menopause, 1998. 5(2): p. 95-101.

168. Visser, M., *et al.*, *Total and sports activity in older men and women: relation with body fat distribution.* Am J Epidemiol, 1997. 145(8): p. 752-61.

169. Hu, J.F., *et al.*, *Bone density and lifestyle characteristics in premenopausal and postmenopausal Chinese women.* Osteoporos Int, 1994. 4(6): p. 288-97.

170. Nicklas, B.J., E.M. Rogus, and A.P. Goldberg, *Exercise blunts declines in lipolysis and fat oxidation after dietary-induced weight loss in obese older women.* Am J Physiol, 1997. 273(1 Pt 1): p. E149-55.

171. Despres, J.P., *et al.*, *Loss of abdominal fat and metabolic response to exercise training in obese women.* Am J Physiol, 1991. 261(2 Pt 1): p. E159-67.

172. Buemann, B. and A. Tremblay, *Effects of exercise training on abdominal obesity and related metabolic complications.* Sports Med, 1996. 21(3): p. 191-212.

173. Lewis, S., *et al.*, *Effects of physical activity on weight reduction in obese middle-aged women.* Am J Clin Nutr, 1976. 29(2): p. 151-6.

174. Sanborn, C.F. and C.M. Jankowski, *Physiologic considerations for women in sport.* Clin Sports Med, 1994. 13(2): p. 315-27.

175. Leon, A.S., *et al.*, *Leisure-time physical activity levels and risk of coronary heart disease and death.* The Multiple Risk Factor Intervention Trial. Jama, 1987. 258(17): p. 2388-95.

176. Ryan, A.S., B.J. Nicklas, and K.E. Dennis, *Aerobic exercise maintains regional bone mineral density during weight loss in postmenopausal women.* J Appl Physiol, 1998. 84(4): p. 1305-10.

177. Kirk, S., *et al.*, *Effect of long-distance running on bone mass in women.* J Bone Miner Res, 1989. 4(4): p. 515-22.

178. van Dam, S., *et al.*, *Effect of exercise on glucose metabolism in postmenopausal women.* Am J Obstet Gynecol, 1988. 159(1): p. 82-6.

179. Baker, C.L., Jr., *Lower extremity problems in female athletes.* J Med Assoc Ga, 1997. 86(3): p. 193-6.

180. Wojtys, E.M., *et al.*, *Association between the menstrual cycle and anterior cruciate ligament injuries in female athletes.* Am J Sports Med, 1998. 26(5): p. 614-9.

181. Liu, S.H., *et al.*, *Estrogen affects the cellular metabolism of the anterior cruciate ligament. A potential explanation for female athletic injury.* Am J Sports Med, 1997. 25(5): p. 704-9.

182. Ryan, A.S., *et al.*, *Resistive training maintains bone mineral density in postmenopausal women.* Calcif Tissue Int, 1998. 62(4): p. 295-9.

183. Morganti, C.M., *et al.*, *Strength improvements with 1 yr of progressive resistance training in older women.* Med Sci Sports Exerc, 1995. 27(6): p. 906-12.

184. Thomas, D.E., J.R. Brotherhood, and J.C. Brand, *Carbohydrate feeding before exercise: effect of glycemic index.* Int J Sports Med, 1991. 12(2): p. 180-6.

185. Thompson, J.L., *et al.*, *Effects of human growth hormone, insulin-like*

growth factor I, and diet and exercise on body composition of obese postmenopausal women. J Clin Endocrinol Metab, 1998. 83(5): p. 1477-84.

186. Svendsen, O.L., et al., *Effects on muscle of dieting with or without exercise in overweight postmenopausal women.* J Appl Physiol, 1996. 80(4): p. 1365-70.

187. Wouassi, D., et al., *Metabolic and hormonal responses during repeated bouts of brief and intense exercise: effects of pre-exercise glucose ingestion.* Eur J Appl Physiol, 1997. 76(3): p. 197-202.

188. Seals, D.R., et al., *Effect of regular aerobic exercise on elevated blood pressure in postmenopausal women.* Am J Cardiol, 1997. 80(1): p. 49-55.

189. Leitzmann, M.F., et al., *The relation of physical activity to risk for symptomatic gallstone disease in men.* Ann Intern Med, 1998. 128(6): p. 417-25.

190. Bass, S., et al., *Exercise before puberty may confer residual benefits in bone density in adulthood: studies in active prepubertal and retired female gymnasts.* J Bone Miner Res, 1998. 13(3): p. 500-7.

191. Kohrt, W.M., A.A. Ehsani, and S.J. Birge, Jr., *HRT preserves increases in bone mineral density and reductions in body fat after a supervised exercise program.* J Appl Physiol, 1998. 84(5): p. 1506-12.

192. Kraemer, R.R., et al., *Effects of hormone replacement on growth hormone and prolactin exercise responses in postmenopausal women.* J Appl Physiol, 1998. 84(2): p. 703-8.

193. Notelovitz, M., et al., *Estrogen therapy and variable-resistance weight training increase bone mineral in surgically menopausal women.* J Bone Miner Res, 1991. 6(6): p. 583-90.

194. Bairey Merz, C.N., et al., *Cardiovascular stress response and coronary artery disease: evidence of an adverse postmenopausal effect in women.* Am Heart J, 1998. 135(5 Pt 1): p. 881-7.

195. Jiang, W., et al., *Mental stress-induced myocardial ischemia and cardiac events.* Jama, 1996. 275(21): p. 1651-6.

196. Gullette, E.C., et al., *Effects of mental stress on myocardial ischemia during daily life.* Jama, 1997. 277(19): p. 1521-6.

197. Matthews, K.A., et al., *Are hostility and anxiety associated with carotid atherosclerosis in healthy postmenopausal women?* Psychosom Med, 1998. 60(5): p. 633-8.

198. Haan, C.K., *What Can Be Done to Prevent Coronary Heart Disease in Women?* Medscape Womens Health, 1996. 1(12): p. 5.

199. Paredes, A., et al., *Stress promotes development of ovarian cysts in rats: the possible role of sympathetic nerve activation.* Endocrine, 1998. 8(3): p. 309-15.

200. Komesaroff, P.A., et al., *Effects of estrogen and estrous cycle on glucocorticoid and catecholamine responses to stress in sheep.* Am J Physiol, 1998. 275(4 Pt 1): p. E671-8.

201. Marucha, P.T., J.K. Kiecolt-Glaser, and M. Favagehi, *Mucosal wound healing is impaired by examination stress.* Psychosom Med, 1998. 60(3): p. 362-5.

202. Kiecolt-Glaser, J.K., *et al., Slowing of wound healing by psychological stress.* Lancet, 1995. 346(8984): p. 1194-6.

203. Virgin, C.E., Jr., *et al., Glucocorticoids inhibit glucose transport and glutamate uptake in hippocampal astrocytes: implications for glucocorticoid neurotoxicity.* J Neurochem, 1991. 57(4): p. 1422-8.

204. Kim, J.J. and K.S. Yoon, *Stress: metaplastic effects in the hippocampus.* Trends Neurosci, 1998. 21(12): p. 505-9.

205. Magarinos, A.M., J.M. Verdugo, and B.S. McEwen, *Chronic stress alters synaptic terminal structure in hippocampus.* Proc Natl Acad Sci U S A, 1997. 94(25): p. 14002-8.

206. Goodman, Y., *et al., Estrogens attenuate and corticosterone exacerbates excitotoxicity, oxidative injury, and amyloid betapeptide toxicity in hippocampal neurons.* J Neurochem, 1996. 66(5): p. 1836-44.

207. Reiter, R.J., *Melatonin and human reproduction.* Ann Med, 1998. 30(1): p. 103-8.

208. Van Cauter, E., *Putative roles of melatonin in glucose regulation.* Therapie, 1998. 53(5): p. 467-72.

209. Scheen, A.J. and E. Van Cauter, *The roles of time of day and sleep quality in modulating glucose regulation: clinical implications.* Horm Res, 1998. 49(3-4): p. 191-201.

210. Spiegel, K, Leproult, R and Van Cauter, E. *Impact of sleep debt on metabolic and endocrine function.* Lancet, 1999 354: p1435-39.

211. Huerta, R., *et al., Symptoms at the menopausal and premenopausal years: their relationship with insulin, glucose, cortisol, FSH, prolactin, obesity and attitudes towards sexuality.* Psychoneuroendocrinology, 1995. 20(8): p. 851-64.

212. Smith, J.A., *et al., Human nocturnal blood melatonin and liver acetylation status.* J Pineal Res, 1991. 10(1): p. 14-7.

213. Frank, S.A., *et al., Effects of aging on glucose regulation during wakefulness and sleep.* Am J Physiol, 1995. 269(6 Pt 1): p. E1006-16.

214. Rosmond, R., *et al., Mental distress, obesity and body fat distribution in middle-aged men.* Obes Res, 1996. 4(3): p. 245-52.

215. Van Cauter, E., *et al., Sleep, awakenings, and insulin-like growth factor-I modulate the growth hormone (GH) secretory response to GH-releasing hormone.* J Clin Endocrinol Metab, 1992. 74(6): p. 1451-9.

216. Grunstein, R.R., *et al., Impact of obstructive sleep apnea and sleepiness on metabolic and cardiovascular risk factors in the Swedish Obese Subjects (SOS) Study.* Int J Obes Relat Metab Disord, 1995. 19(6): p. 410-8.

217. Rosmond, R. and P. Bjorntorp, *Psychiatric ill-health of women and its relationship to obesity and body fat distribution.* Obes Res, 1998. 6(5): p. 338-45.

218. Bray, G.A. and D.A. York, *The MONA LISA hypothesis in the time of leptin.* Recent Prog Horm Res, 1998. 53: p. 95-117.

219. Bylesjo, E.I., K. Boman, and L. Wetterberg, *Obesity treated with phototherapy: four case studies.* Int J Eat Disord, 1996. 20(4): p. 443-46.

220. Borody, W.L., T.E. Brown, and R.S. Boroditsky, *Dietary fat and calcium intakes of menopausal women.* Menopause, 1998. 5(4): p. 230-5.

221. Haines, C.J., et al., *Dietary calcium intake in postmenopausal Chinese women.* Eur J Clin Nutr, 1994. 48(8): p. 591-4.

222. Lau, E.M. and J. Woo, *Nutrition and osteoporosis.* Curr Opin Rheumatol, 1998. 10(4): p. 368-72.

223. Remer, T. and F. Manz, *Potential renal acid load of foods and its influence on urine pH.* J Am Diet Assoc, 1995. 95(7): p: 791-7.

224. Verhoef, P., et al., *Arteriosclerosis,* Thrombosis and Vascular Biology. 17, 1997. 5(989-95).

225. Jacob, R.A., et al., *Moderate folate depletion increases plasma homocysteine and decreases lymphocyte DNA methylation in postmenopausal women.* J Nutr, 1998. 128(7): p. 1204-12.

226. Devine, A., et al., *Effects of zinc and other nutritional factors on insulin-like growth factor I and insulin-like growth factor binding proteins in postmenopausal women.* Am J Clin Nutr, 1998. 68(1): p. 200-6.

227. Kennedy, K.J., T.M. Rains, and N.F. Shay, *Zinc deficiency changes preferred macronutrient intake in subpopulations of Sprague-Dawley outbred rats and reduces hepatic pyruvate kinase gene expression.* J Nutr, 1998. 128(1): p. 43-9.

228. Wood, R.J. and J.J. Zheng, *High dietary calcium intakes reduce zinc absorption and balance in humans.* Am J Clin Nutr, 1997. 65(6): p. 1803-9.

229. Marks, J.W., et al., *Nucleation of biliary cholesterol, arachidonate, prostaglandin E2, and glycoproteins in postmenopausal women.* Gastroenterology, 1997. 112(4): p. 1271-6.

230. Simon, J.A., et al., *Ascorbic acid supplement use and the prevalence of gallbladder disease. Heart & Estrogen-Progestin Replacement Study (HERS) Research Group.* J Clin Epidemiol, 1998. 51(3): p. 257-65.

231. Simon, J.A. and E.S. Hudes, *Serum ascorbic acid and other correlates of gallbladder disease among US adults.* Am J Public Health, 1998. 88(8): p. 1208-12.

232. Simon, J.A., E.S. Hudes, and W.S. Browner, *Serum ascorbic acid and cardiovascular disease prevalence in U.S. adults.* Epidemiology, 1998. 9(3): p. 316-21.

233. Hall, S.L. and G.A. Greendale, *The relation of dietary vitamin C intake to bone mineral density: results from the PEPI study.* Calcif Tissue Int, 1998. 63(3): p. 183-9.

234. Schoenen, J., J. Jacquy, and M. Lenaerts, *Effectiveness of high-dose riboflavin in migraine prophylaxis. A randomized controlled trial.* Neurology, 1998. 50(2): p. 466-70.

235. Kaul, P., *et al., Calculogenic potential of galactose and fructose in relation to urinary excretion of lithogenic substances in vitamin B6 deficient and control rats.* J Am Coll Nutr, 1996. 15(3): p. 295-302.

236. Hansen, C.M., J.E. Leklem, and L.T. Miller, *Vitamin B-6 status indicators decrease in women consuming a diet high in pyridoxine glucoside.* J Nutr, 1996. 126(10): p. 2512-8.

237. Bermond, P., *Therapy of side effects of oral contraceptive agents with vitamin B6.* Acta Vitaminol Enzymol, 1982. 4(1-2): p. 45-54.

238. Graham, I.M., *et al., Plasma homocysteine as a risk factor for vascular disease. The European Concerted Action Project.* Jama, 1997. 277(22): p. 1775-81.

239. Johnston, S.M., *et al., Iron deficiency enhances cholesterol gallstone formation.* Surgery, 1997. 122(2): p. 354-61; discussion 361-2.

240. Steinberg, D., *et al., Beyond cholesterol. Modifications of low-density lipoprotein that increase its atherogenicity.* N Engl J Med, 1989. 320(14): p. 915-24.

241. Boger, R.H., *et al., Dietary L-arginine and alpha-tocopherol reduce vascular oxidative stress and preserve endothelial function in hypercholesterolemic rabbits via different mechanisms.* Atherosclerosis, 1998. 141(1): p. 31-43.

242. Brzozowski, T., *et al., Involvement of endogenous cholecystokinin and somatostatin in gastroprotection induced by intraduodenal fat.* J Clin Gastroenterol, 1998. 27(Suppl 1): p. S125-37.

243. Reckelhoff, J.F., *et al., Long-term dietary supplementation with L-arginine prevents age-related reduction in renal function.* Am J Physiol, 1997. 272(6 Pt 2): p. R1768-74.

244. Daly, J.M., *et al., Immune and metabolic effects of arginine in the surgical patient.* Ann Surg, 1988. 208(4): p. 512-23.

245. Giustina, A., *et al., Arginine blocks the inhibitory effect of hydrocortisone on circulating growth hormone levels in patients with acromegaly.* Metabolism, 1993. 42(5): p. 664-8.

246. Mokdad, A., *et al., The spread of the obesity epidemic in the United States*, 1991-1998. JAMA, Vol.282 (16): p. 1519-1522.

index

order form

Give the gift of great health to your loved ones, friends and colleagues
Check your leading bookstore or order here

fax orders:	**telephone orders:**	**e-mail orders:**	**postal orders:**
(310) 471-9041. *(please send a copy of this form)*	Call 1-(800) 554-3335 toll free or (310) 471-2375 if outside the United States and Canada. *Have your credit card ready.*	orders@ goddessdiet. com	Healthy Life Publications, 264 South La Cienega Blvd., PMB #1233, Beverly Hills, California 90211 USA

Please send _____ copies of *The Goddess Diet* at $17.95 plus $4 shipping per book in the United States (California residents please add $1.48 sales tax per book). Canadian orders must be accompanied by a postal order in U.S. funds. International orders add $9 for shipping.

Please send me information on your other products _____

If you would like to order Female Formula Stress Tabs, Pyridoxal-5-Phosphate or the Goddess Diet Balancer, call 1-800-554-3335 24 hours a day. Operators are waiting for your call.

My check or money order for $_____ is enclosed.
United States $21.95 (outside of California)
                            $23.43 (within California)
Canada $25.00 (US funds)
International $27.00 (US funds)

Please charge my   VISA   MC

Name: _____

Address: _____

City: _____ State: _____ Zip: _____

Phone: _____ E-mail: _____

Card #: _____ Exp date: _____

Signature: _____

Please make your check payable and return to:
Healthy Life Publications
264 S. La Cienega Blvd., PMB #1233, Beverly Hills, California 90211
CALL YOUR CREDIT CARD ORDER TO: 800-554-3335
Fax: 310-471-9041 e-mail: order@goddessdiet.com